医学英语水平考试推荐教材
医学英语新医科课程群系列教材

医学英语基础教程

English for Medical Students and Doctors

主　编　张　洁　高　丽
副主编　王　燕　戴月兰　苏　萍
编　者　王　燕　戴月兰　苏　萍
　　　　王鹏宇　李　雷　李苏明
　　　　陈艳君　张志莉　张　洁
　　　　高　丽

U0361349

南京大学出版社

图书在版编目（CIP）数据

医学英语基础教程 = English for Medical
Students and Doctors / 张洁，高丽主编 . –– 南京：
南京大学出版社，2021.9（2024.6 重印）
　　ISBN 978-7-305-24669-2

　　Ⅰ . ①医… Ⅱ . ①张… ②高… Ⅲ . ①医学 – 英语 –
教材 Ⅳ . ① R

中国版本图书馆 CIP 数据核字（2021）第 125875 号

出版发行　南京大学出版社
社　　址　南京市汉口路22号　　　　　　　邮　编　210093
书　　名　**医学英语基础教程**
　　　　　English for Medical Students and Doctors
主　　编　张　洁　高　丽
责任编辑　裴维维　　　编辑热线　025-83592123

照　　排　南京新华丰制版有限公司
印　　刷　南京凯德印刷有限公司
开　　本　787mm×1092mm　1/16　　印张14.25　　　字数430千
版　　次　2021年9月第1版　2024年6月第3次印刷
ISBN　978-7-305-24669-2
定　　价　77.00元

网　　址：http://www.njupco.com
官方微博：http://weibo.com/njupco
官方微信号：njupress
销售咨询热线：（025）83594756

前 言

　　发展新医科是新时代党和国家对医学教育发展的最新要求。2018 年，教育部颁布了《关于加强医教协同实施卓越医生教育培养计划 2.0 的意见》，全面部署了新医科建设。在新医科背景下高校对医学院校的医学英语课程建设提出了更高的要求。本书正是在此背景下顺应新时代的要求，结合新医科教学计划的特点，全新编写的一本教材。本书编写时注重医学知识与语言知识的有机结合，内容系统全面，可操作性强，适合医学院校医学生，申请成人高等教育本科学士学位的学生以及高等教育自学考试申请学士学位的学生学习使用，可作为临床、全科、儿科、影像、法医、英语等全日制本科专业英语基础课的教材。本书供一学年（两个学期）使用。

　　作为一本专业英语的基础教程，有必要让学习者了解到医学英语的内涵。本书选取了比较常见的六大身体系统，以医学专业内容为主线，"听说读写"四大技能为辅线，全方位多角度地展示医学英语的内涵和外延。本书的设计理念是通过口语和书面语两种不同的文体，展现医学英语在实际工作中的应用，通过"听说读写"保证语言的输入和输出同时进行。

内容简介

　　Warm-up——课前导入，通过形式多样的设计，以问题导入让学生对相关话题进行独立思考或小组讨论，并引出该章的主题。

　　Theme Reading——选取关于人体医学解剖和生理方面的内容，通过主题阅读形式实现用英语学习医学知识。单词表全英文释义，帮助学习者建立英文思维和培养解释医学术语的能力。

　　Medical Terminology——系统学习医学英语构词法知识，通过掌握发音规则、词素分解、英文释义，全方位夯实医学英语词汇知识。

　　Case Study——通过临床病例了解身体系统常见疾病的症状、体征、诊断和治疗等相关信息，掌握基本的病例汇报技巧和语言结构，为临床的实习和带教做好铺垫。

　　Medical Term Extension——通过图片、英文释义、讲解等形式补充相关的临床医学词汇。

　　Medical Conversation——通过医患 / 医医对话的形式熟悉临床工作中提问的技巧和方式，每个单元设置一个主题，从最初的问候打招呼开始，到病人的主诉，采集病史、解释操作与治疗等，覆盖临床问诊的八个方面，了解临床沟通中语言的正确表达方式，充分体现学以致用（本部分可通过扫描单元页二维码获取）。

Writing——通过学习各种体裁的医学应用文，如医学论文的摘要、药品说明书、病例报告、病史等，初步了解医学英语写作的各种体裁和要求，培养学生医学英语写作实践能力。

本书的编写目的在于帮助学习者通过真实的医学语境，触及不同的语言形式，体味不同的语体风格，寄希望能够引起学习者的注意，从而达到触类旁通的目的。由于编者水平有限，不妥之处，敬请读者批评指正。

致学生

掌握医学术语很重要

医学英语课程很重要的一个部分就是医学术语。医学术语（Medical Terminology）是医务工作者之间交流沟通的专业语言，对于医生和护士来说，学习正确的医学术语很重要，医务工作者需要有能力和自信使用专业语言。对于母语不是英语的学习者来说，医学术语的发音、词汇似乎是最棘手的问题，所以本书在 Medical Terminology 部分特别增加了每个医学术语单词的英式发音，目的是通过正确的发音帮助学习者掌握一定的发音规则，例如掌握词根、词缀的常见发音，重读音节和次重读音节的位置，音节划分等，从而更好地记忆医学术语单词。另外，任何词语的学习都不能脱离语言环境，主题阅读（Theme Reading）和病例学习（Case Study）就是一个很好的载体。主题阅读可以帮助学习者用英语学习医学知识；病例学习则帮助学习者了解这些专业语言在临床实际中的应用。

不仅仅是医学术语

医学英语课程通常侧重于医学术语，其实学习医学英语还有更多的内容，不仅仅是医学术语。例如，医务人员工作中经常发现，在谈论病情时，他们的谈话方式需要在日常用语和专业语言之间转换：同事之间追求高效和精确，往往较多使用专业语言，而针对患者医生的表达则需要更易于理解。因此，医生和护士在掌握医学术语的基础上，还需要熟悉病情的大众讲法，这样才能有效地工作。因此，学习者在学习过程中一定要注重英文原文的阅读和普通词汇的积累，这样才能在两种表达方式之间切换自如。本书在建构各个模块内容时，均强调了英文释义的重要性，弱化中文翻译，帮助学习者建立英文思维方式（看图说话和思维导图的制作都是不错的学习方式，建议多多使用）。

案例示范，在两种语言中穿梭

"Cure sometimes, relieve often, comfort always.（有时治愈，常常帮助，总

是安慰。)"这句医学的至理名言提示我们对患者的关怀是医生职能的重要部分。医患沟通作为一项重要的技能正得到越来越多的重视。现在许多医学院都将医患沟通的技能纳入了他们的培训和一些正式考试（如 USMLE）中，要求实习医生通过角色扮演来展示他们的专业态度。在现实诊疗过程中，医生和护士对病人有良好的态度，能够倾听、支持和安抚病人，病人就会感觉更舒服，对医生也更有信心；得到病人的信任后，医生就能从他们的病人那里获得更准确的信息，从而降低出错的风险。医患沟通的技能首先就是语言的沟通能力，医学生和医务工作者应具备与病人沟通的能力，通过非医学术语表达出医务工作者的嘱托。这些技能对于英语非母语人士来说尤其具有挑战性。医学术语似乎更准确，但患者实际上需要医护人员用简洁易懂的方式来表达。这对于英语不是母语的医生和护士来说可能会很困难，因为这需要学习者在现实生活中学习和积累解释医学术语的语言。本书以医患对话中最常见的临床问诊为主线，从内容和语言两个方面进行展示，学习者可以通过角色扮演来练习他们所需要的语言技能，为现实工作和生活做准备。

医学英语学习在专业领域内的继续和提高

医学院校医学生在从事科学研究、论文写作、国际交流时普遍存在着专业英语运用方面的问题。在加强阅读和视听，进行有效的语言输入之外，要学会正确有效的语言输出，从而培养学生医学英语的综合应用能力，尤其是医学英语写作与使用能力，为他们今后在专业领域内的继续与提高打下扎实的语言基础。本书在写作部分，

➢以范例阅读为导入，通过学习各种体裁的医学英语应用文，如 SCI 医学论文、药品说明书、病例报告、病史等，初步了解医学英语写作的各种体裁和结构要求；

➢通过例文实例比照分析，观察文章词语及句式的选用、句子及段落的衔接、篇章的建构、语体风格的转换等，使学生从更高层面上把握语言使用的规律和特点；

➢列举医学英语写作中常见字、词、句、篇章等错误点，通过针对性的讲解和练习进行错误分析，找出错误原因，提高学生对常见错误的敏感性。

写作的过程，是一个由感知到内化的过程，学生需增强语体意识，加强英语思维的能力，并运用语篇知识技能，正确使用语篇衔接手段，从而切实有效地提高英语写作能力。

Contents

Medical Term Extension	Writing
1-1 Positional and Directional Terms 1-2 Planes of the Body	Package Insert—Drug Facts You Should Know
Medical Specialists	A Clinical Case Report
Oral Hygiene	SCI Paper: Title Selection & Title Page
Guidelines on Personal Protective Equipment (PPE)	Medical Abstract (I)
Diagnostic Equipment	Medical Abstract (II)
Basic Surgical Instrument	Tips for Writing the Perfect IMRaD Manuscript
The Metric System	Good Versus Poor Scientific Writing: An Orientation
Common Abbreviations in Medicine	Common Errors in EMP Writing

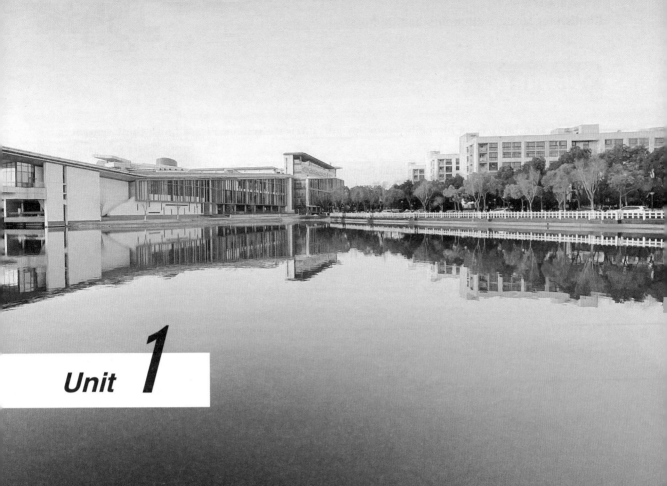

The Human Organism

√ 听力音频
√ 听力文本
√ 课件资源

Warm-up

1. The human body is an incredibly complex and intricate system. Please finish these sentences related to the human body.

(1) The brain is much more active at night than _____.

(2) About 80% of the brain is _____.

(3) The largest internal organ is _____.

(4) The _____ in your stomach is strong enough to dissolve razor blades.

(5) The surface area of a _____ is equal to a tennis court.

(6) Women's hearts beat faster than _____.

(7) _____ is the day of the week when the risk of heart attack is greatest.

(8) Over 90% of diseases are caused or complicated by _____.

(9) You could _____ after removing a large part of your internal organs.

(10) The largest cell in the human body is _____ and the smallest is _____.

2. Choose two interesting facts in Task 1. Discuss the reason(s) behind with your partner.

Theme Reading

The Human Organism

The human body is an amazing structure consisting of nearly 100 trillion cells, the basic unit of life. These cells are organized biologically to eventually form the whole body. To understand the human body, it is necessary to understand how its parts are put together and how they function. The human anatomy and physiology are the study of the structure and function of the human body. In this part, you will have an overall understanding of the human organism.

Objectives

☆ *Define anatomy and explain the importance of understanding the relationship between structure and function.*

☆ *Define physiology and state two major goals of physiology.*

☆ *Describe six levels of organization of the body.*

☆ *List the major organ systems and relate various organs to their respective systems.*

☆ *Describe the major trunk cavities.*

☆ *Define homeostasis and explain why it is important.*

☆ *Define metabolism and the two processes of metabolism.*

Anatomy

Anatomy is the scientific discipline that investigates the structure of the body. The word "anatomy" means dissecting, or cutting apart and separating the parts of the body for study. Anatomy covers a wide range of studies, including the structure of body parts, their microscopic organization, and the processes by which they develop. In addition, anatomy examines the relationship between the structure of a body part and its function. Just as the structure of a hammer makes it well suited for pounding nails, the structure of body parts allows them to perform specific functions effectively. For example, bones can provide strength and support because bone cells surround themselves with a hard, mineralized substance. Understanding the relationship between structure and function makes it easier to understand and appreciate anatomy.

Physiology

Physiology is the scientific discipline that deals with the processes or functions of living things. It is important in physiology to recognize structures as dynamic rather than static, or unchanging. The major goals of physiology are to understand and predict the body's responses to stimuli, and to understand how the body maintains conditions within a narrow range of values in the presence of a continually changing environment.

Physiology is divided according to the **organisms** involved or the levels of organization within a given organism. Human physiology is the study of a specific organism, the human, whereas cellular and systemic physiology are examples of physiology that emphasize specific organizational levels.

Structural and Functional Organization

The body can be studied at six structural levels: the chemical, cell, tissue, organ, organ system, and organism.

Chemical

The structural and functional characteristics of all organisms are determined by their chemical makeup. The chemical level of organization involves interactions among atoms and their combinations into molecules. The function of a molecule is related intimately to its structure. For example, **collagen** molecules are strong, ropelike fibers that give skin structural strength and flexibility. With old age, the structure of collagen changes and the skin becomes fragile and is torn more easily.

Cell

Cells are the basic structural and functional units of organisms, such as plants and animals. Molecules can combine to form organelles (Figure 1-1), which are the small structures that make up cells. For example, the nucleus contains the cell's hereditary information and mitochondria manufacture **adenosine triphosphate** (ATP), which is a molecule used by cells for a source of energy. Although cell types differ in their structure and function, they have many characteristics in common. Knowledge of these characteristics and their variations is essential to a basic understanding of anatomy and physiology.

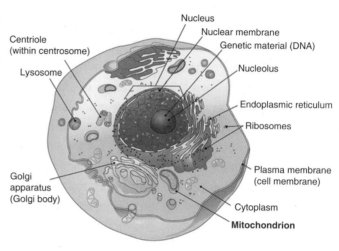

Figure 1-1 A typical animal cell

Tissue

A tissue is a group of similar cells and the materials surrounding them. The characteristics of the cells and surrounding materials determine the functions of the tissue. The many tissues that make up the body are classified into four primary tissue types: **epithelial**, connective, muscular and nervous.

Organ

An organ is composed of two or more tissue types that together perform one or more common functions. The urinary bladder, skin, stomach, eye and heart are examples of organs.

Organ system

An organ system is a group of organs classified as a unit because of a common function or set of functions. For example, the **urinary** system consists of the kidneys, **ureters**, urinary **bladder** and **urethra**. The kidneys produce urine, which is transported by the ureters to the urinary bladder, where it is stored until eliminated from the body by passing through the urethra. Usually the body is considered to have 11 major organ systems: **integumentary**, **skeletal**, muscular, **lymphatic**, **respiratory**, **digestive**, nervous, **endocrine**, **cardiovascular**, urinary and **reproductive**.

The coordinated activity of the organ systems is necessary for normal function. For example, the digestive system takes in and processes food, which is carried by the blood of the cardiovascular system to the cells of the other systems. These cells use the food and produce waste products that are carried by the blood to the kidneys of the urinary system, which removes waste products from the blood. Because the organ systems are so interrelated, dysfunction of one organ system can have profound effects on other systems. For example, a heart attack can result in inadequate circulation of blood. Consequently, the organs of other systems, such as the brain and kidneys, can **malfunction**.

Organism

An organism is any living thing considered as a whole, whether composed of one cell, such as a bacterium, or trillions of cells, such as a human. The human organism is a complex of organ systems that are mutually dependent on one another.

Body Cavities

The organs that comprise most of the body systems are located in four cavities: **cranial**, **spinal**, **thoracic**, and **abdominopelvic**. The cranial and spinal cavities are within a larger region known as the **dorsal** (posterior) cavity. The thoracic and abdominopelvic cavities are found in the **ventral** (anterior) cavity. (Figure 1-2)

The dorsal cavity contains the brain and spinal cord: The brain is in the cranial cavity and the spinal cord is in the spinal cavity. The **diaphragm** divides the ventral cavity into two parts: the upper thoracic and lower abdominopelvic cavities.

The central area of the thoracic cavity is called the **mediastinum**. It lies between the lungs and extends from the **sternum** (breast bone) to the **vertebrae** of the back. The **esophagus**, **bronchi**, lungs, **trachea**, **thymus** gland and

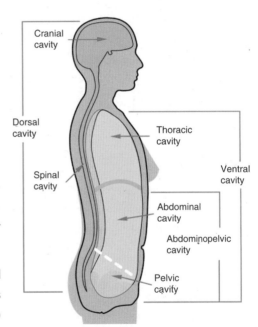

Figure 1-2 Body cavities

heart are located in the thoracic cavity. The heart itself is enclosed by a smaller cavity, called the **pericardial** cavity.

The thoracic cavity is further subdivided into two pleural cavities: The left lung is surrounded by the left cavity; the right lung is surrounded by the right cavity. Each lung is covered with a thin membrane called the **pleura**.

The abdominopelvic cavity is actually one large cavity with no separation between the abdomen and pelvis. To avoid confusion, this cavity is usually referred to separately as the abdominal cavity and the pelvic cavity. The abdominal cavity contains the stomach, liver, **gallbladder**, **pancreas**, spleen, small **intestine**, **appendix** and part of the large intestine. The kidneys are close to but behind the abdominal cavity. The urinary bladder, reproductive organs, **rectum**, remainder of the large intestine and appendix are in the pelvic cavity. (Figures 1-3, 1-4)

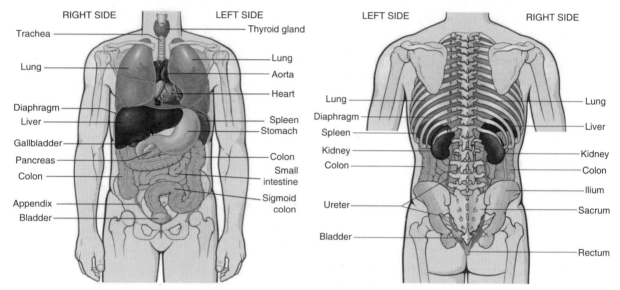

Figure 1-3 Organs of the abdominopelvic and thoracic cavities, anterior view

Figure 1-4 Organs of the abdominopelvic and thoracic cavities, posterior view

Smaller Cavities

In addition to the cranial cavity, the skull also contains several smaller cavities. The eyes, eyeball muscles, **optic** nerves and **lacrimal** (tear) ducts are within the **orbital** cavity. The **nasal** cavity contains the parts that form the nose. The oral or **buccal** cavity encloses the teeth and tongue.

Body Processes

Homeostasis

Homeostasis is the ability of the body to regulate its' internal environment within narrow limits. Homeostasis is essential to survival: many of our body's systems are concerned with maintaining the internal environment. Examples of homeostasis controls are blood sugar levels, body temperature, heart rate and the fluid environment of the cells.

Homeostasis works on a negative feedback mechanism. An example of how it operates is seen in maintaining our body temperature. Our normal body temperature is 98.6°F. Outside, on a very hot summer day, our body temperature rises. The **hypothalamus** in the brain detects this and sends signals to various organs and we start to sweat (sweating is a cooling process). As water is excreted by the sweat glands on the skin, it evaporates (**evaporation** is a cooling mechanism). In addition, our blood vessels dilate to bring blood near the skin's surface to dissipate body heat. If we go outside on a cold day and our body temperature falls below 98.6 degrees, the hypothalamus of the brain detects this and sends signals to muscles causing us to shiver, which raises the body temperature (increased muscle activity produces heat). In addition, the hypothalamus sends signals to the blood vessels, causing them to constrict, which reduces blood flow near the surface, which conserves body heat.

Metabolism

The functional activities of cells that result in growth, repair, energy release, use of food and secretions are combined under the heading of metabolism. Metabolism consists of two processes that are opposite to each other: anabolism and catabolism. **Anabolism** is the building up of complex materials from simpler ones such as food and oxygen. **Catabolism** is the breaking down and changing of complex substances into simpler ones, with a release of energy and carbon dioxide. The sum of all the chemical reactions within a cell is therefore called metabolism.

Vocabulary

abdominopelvic [ˌæbˌdɒmɪnəʊˈpelvɪk]　of or pertaining to the abdomen and (the cavity of) the pelvis

adenosine [əˈdenəsiːn]　(biochemistry) a nucleoside that is a structural component of nucleic acids; it is present in all living cells in a combined form as a constituent of DNA, RNA, ADP, ATP and AMP

anabolism [əˈnæbəˌlɪzəm]　synthesis of more complex substances from simpler ones

anatomy [əˈnætəmi]　the branch of morphology that deals with the structure of animals

appendix [əˈpendɪks]　(pl. appendices or appendixes) a vestigial process that extends from the lower end of the cecum and that resembles a small pouch

bladder [ˈblædə(r)]　a distensible membranous sac (usually containing liquid or gas)

bronchus [ˈbrɒŋkəs]　(pl. bronchi) either of the two main branches of the trachea

buccal [ˈbʌkəl]　of or relating to or toward the cheek

cardiovascular [ˌkɑːdiəʊˈvæskjələ(r)]　of or pertaining to or involving the heart and blood vessels

catabolism [kəˈtæbəlizəm]　breakdown of more complex substances into simpler ones with release of energy

collagen [ˈkɒlədʒən]　a fibrous scleroprotein in bone, cartilage, tendon and other connective tissue

cranial [ˈkreɪniəl]　of or relating to the cranium which encloses the brain

diaphragm [ˈdaɪəfræm]　a muscular partition separating the abdominal and thoracic cavities

digestive [daɪˈdʒestɪv]　relating to or having the power to cause or promote digestion

dorsal [ˈdɔːsl]　belonging to or on or near the back or upper surface of an animal or organ or part

endocrine [ˈendəʊkraɪn]　of or belonging to endocrine glands or their secretions

epithelial [ˌepɪˈθiːliəl]　of or belonging to the epithelium

esophagus [ɪˈsɒfəgəs]　the passage between the pharynx and the stomach

evaporation [ɪˌvæpəˈreɪʃn]　the process of becoming a vapor

gallbladder [ˈgɔːlblædə]　a muscular sac that stores and concentrates bile until needed for digestion

homeostasis [ˌhəʊmiəʊˈsteɪsɪs] metabolic equilibrium actively maintained by several complex biological mechanisms that operate via the autonomic nervous system to offset disrupting changes

hypothalamus [ˌhaɪpəˈθæləməs] a basal part of the diencephalon governing autonomic nervous system

integumentary [ɪnˌtegjʊˈmentəri] of or relating to the integument

intestine [ɪnˈtestɪn] the part of the alimentary canal between the stomach and the anus

lacrimal [ˈlækrɪml] of or relating to tears

lymphatic [lɪmˈfætɪk] of or relating to or produced by lymph

malfunction [ˌmælˈfʌŋkʃn] a failure to function normally

mediastinum [ˌmiːdɪəsˈtaɪnəm] (pl. mediastina) the part of the thoracic cavity between the lungs that contains the heart, aorta, esophagus, trachea and thymus

metabolism [məˈtæbəlɪzəm] the organic processes (in a cell or organism) that are necessary for life

mitochondrion [ˌmaɪtəˈkɒndrɪən] (pl. mitochondria) an organelle containing enzymes responsible for producing energy

nasal [ˈneɪzəl] of or in or relating to the nose

optic [ˈɒptɪk] of or relating to or resembling the eye; relating to or using sight

orbital [ˈɔːbɪtl] of or relating to the eye socket

organism [ˈɔːgənɪzəm] a living thing that has (or can develop) the ability to act or function independently

pancreas [ˈpæŋkrɪəs] a large elongated exocrine gland located behind the stomach which secretes pancreatic juice and insulin

pericardial [perɪˈkɑːdɪəl] located around the heart or relating to or affecting the pericardium

physiology [ˌfɪziˈɒlədʒi] the branch of the biological sciences dealing with the functioning of organisms

pleural [ˈplʊərə] of or relating to the pleura or the walls of the thorax

rectum [ˈrektəm] (pl. recta or rectums) the terminal section of the alimentary canal, from the sigmoid flexure to the anus

reproductive [ˌriːprəˈdʌktɪv] producing new life or offspring

respiratory [ˈrespərətəri; rɪˈspaɪə-] pertaining to respiration

skeletal [ˈskelətl] of or relating to or forming or attached to a skeleton

spinal [ˈspaɪnl] of or relating to the spine or spinal cord

sternum [ˈstɜːnəm] the flat bone that articulates with the clavicles and the first seven pairs of ribs

thoracic [θɔːˈræsɪk] of or relating to the chest or thorax

thymus [ˈθaɪməs] a ductless glandular organ at the base of the neck that produces lymphocytes and aids in producing immunity

trachea [treɪkɪə] (pl. tracheae or tracheas) windpipe, the membranous tube with cartilaginous rings that conveys inhaled air from the larynx to the bronchi

triphosphate [traɪˈfɒsfeɪt] a salt or acid that contains three phosphate groups

ureter [jʊəˈriːtə] either of a pair of thick-walled tubes that carry urine from the kidney to the urinary bladder

urethra [jʊəˈriːθrə] duct through which urine is discharged in most mammals and which serves as the male genital duct

urinary [ˈjʊərɪnəri] of or relating to the function or production or secretion of urine; of or relating to the urinary system of the body

ventral [ˈventrəl] toward or on or near the belly

vertebra [ˈvɜːtɪbrə] (pl. vertebrae) one of the bony segments of the spinal column

Task 1

Directions: *Select the letter of the choice that best completes the statement or answers the question.*

(1) Which of the following is within the scope of the gross anatomy?
    A. The processes of the lungs.   B. The structure of the cell.
    C. The functions of the liver.   D. The size and shape of the kidney.

(2) The study of the function of each body part and how the functions of the various body parts coordinate to form a complete living organism is called _____.
    A. anatomy   B. physiology   C. histology   D. microbiology

(3) The molecule which is the major source of energy for cellular reactions is called _____.
    A. adenosine triphosphate B. organelle   C. mitochondrion   D. nucleus

(4) A part of an organism consisting of an aggregate of cells having a similar structure and function is called _____.
    A. a cell   B. a tissue   C. an organ   D. an organ system

(5) The system that deals with the skin and its appendages is called _____.
    A. the skeletal system   B. the reproductive system
    C. the integumentary system   D. the digestive system

(6) The brain and spinal cord are located in _____.
    A. the dorsal cavity   B. the ventral cavity   C. the spinal cavity   D. the cranial cavity

(7) The muscular partition separating the abdominal and thoracic cavities is called _____.
    A. the sternum   B. the mediastinum   C. the diaphragm   D. the rectum

(8) The breakdown of more complex substances into simpler ones with release of energy and carbon dioxide is called _____.
    A. anabolism   B. catabolism   C. metabolism   D. evaporation

(9) The scientific name for the chest cavity is _____.
    A. the cervical cavity   B. the ventral cavity   C. the thoracic cavity   D. the pelvic cavity

(10) _____ is the state of steady internal physical and chemical conditions maintained by living systems.
    A. Metastasis   B. Metabolism   C. Hemostasis   D. Homeostasis

Task 2

Directions: *Place the following organs in their proper body cavity.*

(1) brain   _____ cavity
(2) spinal cord   _____ cavity
(3) esophagus   _____ cavity
(4) thymus gland   _____ cavity

(5) lung   _____ cavity

(6) heart   _____ cavity

(7) liver   _____ cavity

(8) pancreas   _____ cavity

(9) small intestine   _____ cavity

(10) tongue   _____ cavity

(11) urinary bladder   _____ cavity

(12) appendix   _____ cavity

Task 3

Directions: *List the main organs or components of the systems.*

Systems	Main components
The integumentary system	
The musculoskeletal system	
The respiratory system	
The digestive system	
The nervous system	
The endocrine system	
The cardiovascular system	
The urinary system	
The male reproductive system	
The female reproductive system	

Task 4

Directions: *What body systems do you see in the pictures? Write underneath.*

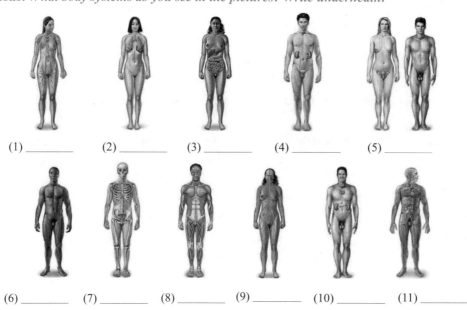

(1) _____   (2) _____   (3) _____   (4) _____   (5) _____

(6) _____   (7) _____   (8) _____   (9) _____   (10) _____   (11) _____

Medical Terminology

The word-formation processes of English include affixation, compounding, conversion, blending, backformation, clipping, acronym, coinage, etc. Affixation is the most commonly used word-formation process in English medical terminology.

Affixation (also called derivation) refers to the formation of words by means of affixes (prefix and suffix). It includes prefixation and suffixation. Prefixation is a morphological process whereby a prefix is attached to the front of a stem. Usually, prefixation tends to be semantically oriented, that is, the process does not generally change the word class of the stem, but only modifies its meaning.

There are prefixes such as negative prefixes (e.g. a-, in-, non-), reversative prefixes (e.g. de-, un-, dis-), pejorative prefixes (e.g. mal-, mis-), "degree or size" prefixes (e.g. hyper-, hypo-, sub-, extra-), "orientation and attitude" prefixes (e.g. contra-, anti-, pro), locative prefixes (e.g. inter-, intra-, trans-), "time and order" prefixes (e.g. post-, re-, pre), number prefixes (e.g. bi-, uni-, tri-), miscellaneous prefixes (e.g. ultra-). However, there are an increasing number of class-changing prefixes in present-day English such as asleep, encourage, which only make up an insignificant number in the contemporary vocabulary.

Suffixation is a morphological process where a suffix is attached to the end of a stem. Suffixes tend to change the grammatical function of stems, in other words, to change the word class, which can be classified into the followings: nominal suffixes (e.g. -ment, -tion, -ism), verbal suffixes (e.g. -ate, -fy, -en, -ize), adjectival suffixes (e.g. -ful, -ish, -al, -ous) and adverbial suffixes (e.g. -ly, -ward, -wise). In English medical terminology, there is still another group of suffixes which can change the meaning of the word. For example, "-itis" is a most commonly-used suffix meaning inflammation and "-oma" means tumor or morbid growth. If we add "-itis" or "-oma" to the word root hepat(o)- (the liver), we can get the word hepatitis (inflammation of the liver) and hepatoma (carcinoma of the liver).

Nominal Endings			
Suffixes	Terminology	Term Analysis	Definition
act, process, condition			
-a	aerobia [eəˈrəʊbɪə] placenta [pləˈsentə]	aer(o)=air placent(o) =placenta	
-e	lymphocyte [ˈlɪmfəsaɪt] isotope [ˈaɪsətəʊp]	lymph(o)=lymph cyt(o)=cell is(o)=equal top(o)=location	
-is	cutis [ˈkju:tɪs] prognosis [prɒgˈnəʊsɪs]	cut(i)=skin pro-=before gnos=knowledge	

(to be continued)

-on	neuron [ˈnjʊərɒn]	neur(o)=nerve	
	colon [ˈkəʊlən]	col(o)=colon	
-um	cerebrum [ˈserəbrəm]	cerebr(o)=cerebrum	
	pericardium [ˌperɪˈkɑːdɪəm]	peri-=surrounding cardi(o)=heart	
-us	thrombus [ˈθrɒmbəs]	thromb(o)=blood clot	
	nucleus [ˈnjuːklɪəs]	nucle(o)=nucleus	
-y	biopsy [ˈbaɪɒpsi]	bi(o)=living thing ops(o)=vision	
	physiology [ˌfɪziˈɒlədʒi]	physi(o)=nature log(o)=speech	
Adjective Endings			
pertaining to			
-ac	cardiac [ˈkɑːdɪæk]	cardi(o)=heart	
-aceous	sebaceous [sɪˈbeɪʃəs]	seb(o)=oily, fatty	
-al	buccal [ˈbʌkəl]	bucc(o)=cheek	
-ar	muscular [ˈmʌskjələ(r)]	muscul(o)=muscle	
-ary	biliary [ˈbɪliəri]	bil(i)=bile	
-eal	esophageal [iːˌsɒfəˈdʒiːəl]	esophag(o)=food tube	
-ic	optic [ˈɒptɪk]		
-ory	respiratory [ˈrespərətəri; riˈspaɪə-]	re-=again spir(o)=breath -at(e)=verbal ending	
-ous	infectious [ɪnˈfekʃəs]		
	mucous [ˈmjuːkəs]		
Diminutive Endings			
small, little			
-cul(e), -cle	ventricular [venˈtrɪkjʊlə] corpuscle [ˈkɔːpʌsl] vesicle [ˈvesɪkl]	vesic(o)=sac	
-ell	organelle [ˌɔːgəˈnel] circellus [sɜːˈseləs]		
-ill(us, a, um)	capillary [kəˈpɪləri] bacillus [bəˈsɪləs]	bac(i)=rod	
-ol	arteriole [ɑːˈtɪəriəʊl] bronchiole [ˈbrɒŋkɪəʊl]	arteri(o)=artery bronch(i)=bronchus	
-ul(e)	venule [ˈvenjuːl] lobule [ˈlɒbjuːl]	ven(o)=vein lob(o)=lobe	
Diseased Condition			
abnormal or pathological condition			
-esis	diuresis [ˌdaɪjʊəˈriːsɪs]	ur(o)=urine	

(to be continued)

-ia	leukemia [luːˈkiːmiə]	leuk(o)=white	
-iasis	lithiasis [lɪˈθaɪəsɪs]	lith(o)=stone	
-osis	acidosis [ˌæsɪˈdəʊsɪs] necrosis [neˈkrəʊsɪs]	necr(o)=death	
enzyme			
-ase	lipase [ˈlaɪpeɪz] oxidase [ˈɒksɪdeɪz]	lip(o)=fat, lipid ox(i)=oxygen	
sugar			
-ose	fructose [ˈfrʌktəʊs] glucose [ˈgluːkəʊs]	fruct(o)=fruit	
agent			
-in, -ine	insulin [ˈɪnsjəlɪn] epinephrine [ˌepɪˈnefrɪn] immunoglobulin [ˌɪmjənəʊˈglɒbjʊlən]	insul(o)=islet nephr(o)=kidney immun(o)=immunity	
inflammation			
-itis	arthritis [ɑːˈθraɪtɪs] hepatitis [ˌhepəˈtaɪtɪs]	arthr(o)=joint hepat(o)=liver	
tumor			
-oma	adenoma [ˌædiˈnəʊmə] hematoma [ˌhiːməˈtəʊmə]	aden(o)=gland hemat(o)=blood	
resembling			
-oid	adenoid [ˈædɪnɔɪd] cystoid [ˈsɪstɔɪd]	cyst(o)=sac, bladder	
name of a science			
-ics	genetics [dʒəˈnetɪks] pediatrics [ˌpiːdɪˈætrɪks]	genet(o)=heredity ped(i)=child	
an expert of a profession			
-ician	physician [fɪˈzɪʃn] pediatrician [ˌpiːdɪəˈtrɪʃn]	physi(o)=nature	
practitioner of a profession			
-ist	dentist [ˈdentɪst] physiologist [ˌfɪziˈɒlədʒɪst]	dent(o)=tooth	
act, process; state, condition; abnormal state or condition			
-ism	embolism [ˈembəlɪzəm] rheumatism [ˈruːmətɪzəm]		

Vocabulary Study

Task 1

Directions: *Underline the suffixes in the following terms and explain these suffixes.*

(1) adenosine _____   (2) urinary _____

(3) metabolism _____ (4) organism _____

(5) epithelial _____ (6) organelle _____

(7) dorsal _____ (8) adrenaline _____

(9) intracranial _____ (10) gastroscope _____

(11) transaminase _____ (12) pharmacist _____

(13) obstetrician _____ (14) cardiovascular _____

(15) sternum _____ (16) homeostasis _____

(17) thoracic _____ (18) angioplasty _____

(19) mediastinum _____ (20) circulation _____

Task 2

Directions: *Explain the meanings of the following terms related to the nerve and underline the strong part of each word where there are two or more syllables. Pay attention to the suffixes.*

(1) neuron _____

(2) neural _____

(3) neurology _____

(4) neurologist _____

(5) neuritis _____

(6) neuralgia _____

(7) neuroma _____

(8) neuroid _____

(9) neurogenic _____

(10) neurogenesis _____

(11) neurotoxin _____

(12) neurotubule _____

(13) neurosis _____

(14) neuropathy _____

(15) neurocyte _____

(16) neurolysis _____

(17) neurectomy _____

(18) neurotomy _____

(19) neurotic _____

(20) neuraminidase _____

Case Study 1-1

Emergency Care

During a triathlon, paramedics responded to a scene with multiple patients involved in a serious bicycle accident. B.R., a 20-YO woman, lost control of her bike while descending a hill at approximately 40 mph. As she fell, two other cyclists collided with her, sending all three crashing to the ground.

At the scene, B.R. reported pain in her head, back, chest, and leg. She also had numbness and tingling in her legs and feet. Other injuries included a cut on her face and on her right arm and an obvious deformity to both her shoulder and knee. She had slight difficulty breathing.

The paramedic did a rapid cephalocaudal assessment and immobilized B.R.'s neck in a cervical collar. She was secured on a backboard and given oxygen. After her bleeding was controlled and her injured extremities were immobilized, she was transported to the nearest emergency department.

During transport, the paramedic in charge radioed ahead to provide a prehospital report to the charge nurse. His report included the following information: occipital and frontal head pain; laceration to right temple, superior, and anterior to right ear; lumbar pain; bilateral thoracic pain on inspiration at midclavicular line on the right and midaxillary line on the left; dull aching pain of the posterior proximal right thigh; bilateral paresthesia (numbness and tingling) of distal lower legs circumferentially; varus (knock-knee) adduction deformity of left knee; and posterior displacement deformity of left shoulder.

At the hospital, the emergency department physician ordered radiographs for B.R. Before the procedure, the radiology technologist positioned a lead gonadal shield centered on the midsagittal line above B.R.'s symphysis pubis to protect her ovaries from unnecessary irradiation by the primary beam. The technologist knew that gonadal shielding is important for female patients undergoing imaging of the lumbar spine, sacroiliac joints, acetabula, pelvis, and kidneys. Shields should not be used for any examination in which an acute abdominal condition is suspected.

Task 3

Directions: *Find ten words in the case study with prefixes, underline the prefixes and write down the meaning of the prefixes.*

Word with Prefix	Meaning of the Prefix

Task 4

Directions: *Find words in the case study with suffixes that mean "pertaining to", and write down both the suffix and the word that contains it.*

Suffix	Word

Case Study 1-2

R.S.'s Self-Diagnosis

Chief Complaint:

R.S. is a second-year medical student. Recently, he finds that he is always tired and unable to focus in class. He decides to self-diagnose and begins with a review of systems (ROS). He notes that he is not having any cardiovascular, lymphatic, or respiratory system symptoms, such as tissue swelling, coughing, or shortness of breath. He also has not noticed any changes in urinary system functions. He realizes that he has gained some weight recently and has also been a little constipated but has no other problems with his digestive system. He rules out anything concerning his musculoskeletal system because he has no muscle cramps, joint pain, or weakness. He thinks his skin is drier than usual. He worries that this is an integumentary system sign of hypothyroidism and becomes concerned about his endocrine system function. Unable to perform any imaging studies or lab tests on his own, he makes an appointment to see a campus health services physician.

Examination:

R.S. tells the doctor he feels he has a metabolic disorder. He thinks he might have an adenoma, a glandular tumor that is disrupting homeostasis, his normal metabolic state. The doctor takes a complete history and orders various blood tests to assist with the diagnosis. He completes a physical examination that reveals no abnormalities.

Clinical Course:

The blood glucose levels, complete blood count (CBC), and thyroid function tests are all normal. Nothing in the tests indicates anything physically wrong with the patient. There is no indication that any further cytologic or histologic tests are necessary. The doctor tells R.S. that he is sleep-deprived from all his studying and that his weight gain can be explained by his poor food choices in the university cafeteria. In addition, the doctor advises R.S. to schedule some exercise into his daily routine. Lastly, he reminds R.S. that although he is studying to be a doctor, self-diagnosis at this point in his career could be inaccurate and could cause undue anxiety.

Task 5

Directions: *Select the best answer to the question based on the information provided in Case 1-2.*

(1) On review of systems, R.S. rules out problems with all the following systems EXCEPT _____.
   A. the musculoskeletal system   B. the lymphatic system
   C. the digestive system   D. the endocrine system

(2) The symptom "shortness of breath" usually indicates a problem with _____.
   A. the integumentary system or the digestive system
   B. the cardiovascular system or the respiratory system
   C. the skeletal system or the muscular system
   D. the urinary system or the reproductive system

(3) The opposite of "hypothyroidism" is _____.
   A. parathyroid   B. hypertension   C. hyperthyroidism   D. hypothermia

(4) The word "adenoma" has a suffix meaning _____.
   A. tumor   B. inflammation   C. gland   D. disease

(5) The campus health services physician orders various _____ to assist with the diagnosis.
   A. cytologic tests   B. histologic tests   C. blood tests   D. radioisotope studies

(6) R.S. has the following symptoms EXCEPT _____.
   A. fatigue   B. dry skin   C. weight loss   D. impaired concentration

Medical Term Extension

Positional and Directional Terms

In describing the location or direction of a given point in the body, it is always assumed that the subject is in the anatomic position, that is, upright, with face front, arms at the sides with palms forward and feet parallel, as shown in Figure 1-5.

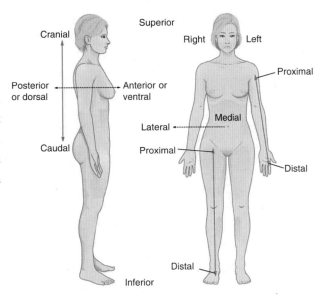

Figure 1-5 Directional terms

Location	Relationship
Anterior/Ventral	Front side of the body. Example: *The forehead is on the anterior side of the body.*
Posterior/Dorsal	The back side of the body. Example: *The back of the head is posterior (dorsal) to the face.*
Deep/Internal	Away from the surface. Example: *The stab wound penetrated deep into the abdomen.*
Superficial/External	On the surface. Example: *Superficial veins can be viewed through the skin.*
Proximal	Near the point of attachment to the trunk or near the beginning of a structure. Example: *The proximal end of the thigh bone (femur) joins with the hip socket.*
Distal	Far from the point of attachment to the trunk or far from the beginning of a structure. Example: *At its distal end, the femur joins with the knee.*
Superior	Above another structure. Example: *The head lies superior to the neck.*
Inferior	Below another structure. Example: *The feet are at the inferior part of the body. They are inferior to the knees.*
Cephalic/Cranial	Cephalic (pertaining to the head) also means above another structure.
Caudal	Pertaining to the tail, or to the lower portion of the body, also means away from the head or below another structure.
Medial	Pertaining to the middle, or nearer the medial plane of the body. Example: *When in the anatomic position (palms of the hands facing outward), the fifth (little) finger is medial.*
Lateral	Pertaining to the side. Example: *When in the anatomic position (palms of the hands facing outward), the thumb is lateral.*
Supine	Lying on the back. Example: *The patient lies supine during an examination of the abdomen. (The face is up in the supine position.)*
Prone	Lying on the belly. Example: *The backbones are examined with the patient in a prone position. (The patient lies on his or her stomach in the prone position.)*

Planes of the Body

A plane is an imaginary flat surface. Organs appear in different relationships to one another according to the plane of the body in which they are viewed.

Plane	Location
Frontal/Coronal plane	Vertical plane dividing the body or structure into anterior and posterior portions. Example: *A common chest X-ray view is a PA (posteroanterior—viewed from back to front) view, which is in the frontal (coronal) plane.*

(to be continued)

Sagittal/Lateral plane	Lengthwise vertical plane dividing the body or structure into right and left sides. Example: *The midsagittal plane divides the body into right and left halves.* *A lateral (side-to-side) chest X-ray film is taken in the sagittal plane.*
Transverse/Axial plane	Horizontal (cross-sectional) plane running across the body parallel to the ground. This cross-sectional plane divides the body or structure into upper and lower portions. Example: *A CT (computed tomography) scan is one of a series of X-ray pictures taken in the transverse (axial or cross-sectional) plane.*

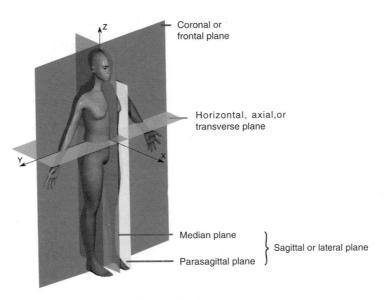

Figure 1-6 Planes of the body

Task 6

Directions: *Label the picture below.*

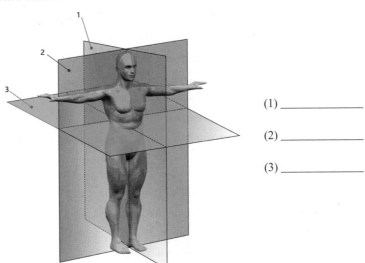

(1) _____

(2) _____

(3) _____

Task 7

Directions: Select from the following medical terms to complete the sentences below.

distal	frontal (coronal)	inferior (caudal)	lateral
proximal	superior (cephalic)	transverse (axial)	midsagittal

(1) The kidney lies _____ to the spinal cord. (Hint: to the side of)

(2) The _____ end of the thigh bone (femur) joins with the kneecap (patella).

(3) The _____ plane divides the body into an anterior and a posterior portion.

(4) The diaphragm lies _____ to the organs in the thoracic cavity.

(5) The _____ plane divides the body into right and left halves.

(6) The _____ end of the upper arm bone (humerus) is at the shoulder.

(7) The _____ plane divides the body into upper and lower portions.

(8) The pharynx is located _____ to the esophagus.

Writing

Package Insert
—Drug Facts You Should Know

Drug labels for over-the-counter and prescription medicines provide important information on safe and proper medication use. There are two kinds of drug labels: over-the-counter drug labels—also called Drug Facts—and prescription drug labels, which include many pages of safety information, such as pharmacy information sheets, medication guides and prescribing information.

Over the Counter Drug Label

Over-the-counter, or OTC, drugs are medications that don't require a prescription. Manufacturers print drug labels called Drug Facts directly on OTC drug product packages. These labels are short and simple and typically have six main parts. Some labels include a seventh section with a phone number to call if you have questions or comments.

The Drug Facts panel on an over-the-counter med lets you know how to take it, what's in it, and how it might make you feel. But the way that info is written can make it tricky to understand. Here's how to make sense of drug labels so you can avoid common, possibly dangerous mistakes.

Active Ingredient and Purpose

Find this info at the top of the label on over-the-counter meds. It's the ingredient in the medicine that treats a symptom, along with the type of medication it is, like "antihistamine" or "pain reliever". It also tells you how much of the drug is in each dose. Check this to make sure you don't take other drugs with the same ingredient and to understand what the product will do for you.

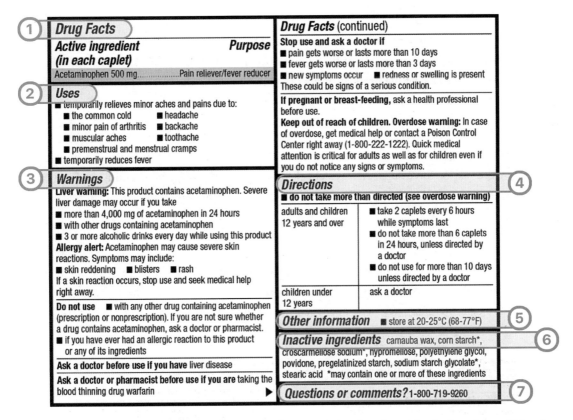

(1) Drug Facts	Drug Facts (continued)
Active ingredient *Purpose* **(in each caplet)** Acetaminophen 500 mg..................Pain reliever/fever reducer	**Stop use and ask a doctor if** ■ pain gets worse or lasts more than 10 days ■ fever gets worse or lasts more than 3 days ■ new symptoms occur ■ redness or swelling is present These could be signs of a serious condition.

The Drug Facts label for the over-the-counter drug acetaminophen, known by the brand name Tylenol.

Uses

This section gives you a snapshot of the symptoms or diseases that the drug can treat. For example, a pain-reliever label might say it eases toothaches, headaches, joint pain, and menstrual cramps. Always check this part when you buy a new medication to make sure it will do what you need it to do.

Warnings

This is one of the most important parts of the drug label, and it's usually the largest. It gives you safety details about the medicine. You'll find four things here: who shouldn't take the drug, when you should stop using it, when to call your doctor, and side effects you might have. It can help you check if it's not safe to take with some health conditions or other medications.

Directions

Check this part carefully. It tells you how much of the drug to take and how often to take it, called the dosage. For example, it may say to take two tablets every 4 to 6 hours. Never take more than the label says without talking to your doctor. The directions are grouped by age, so you know how much you or your child can use. You'll also get details about the maximum amount you should take in 1 day.

Other Information

Heat and humidity can sometimes damage medications, so keeping them in your bathroom or in a car when the weather's warm may not be a good idea. This part of the label will tell you the right temperature range for storing the product. It also reminds you to make sure the package's safety seal hasn't been broken before you use it, which could be a sign of tampering.

Inactive Ingredients

These are the ingredients in a drug that don't directly treat your symptoms. They might be preservatives, dyes, or flavorings. Always check this section if you or your child has food or dye allergies. Keep in mind that different brands of the same kind of drug may have different inactive ingredients.

Prescription Drug Label

Prescription drug labels are more complicated than OTC drug labels. The FDA doesn't regulate the labels from pharmacies. Warning information printed or placed on the bottle as stickers may vary depending on the pharmacy. The approved prescribing information—also called professional

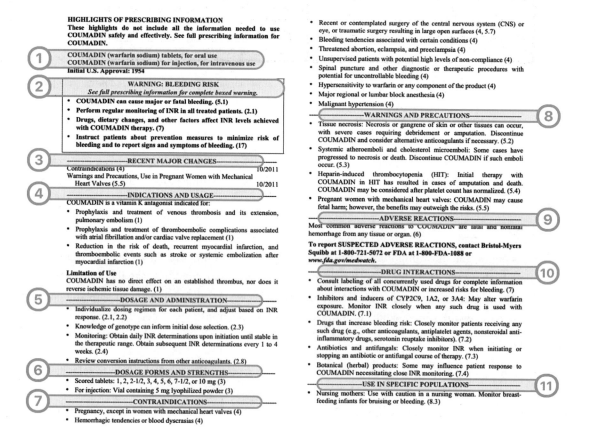

labeling, package insert and prescribing information—is the actual prescription drug label. The prescribing information is several pages long, and it's intended to help providers properly prescribe the medication. The highlights section is a half-page summary of the information that health care practitioners most commonly refer to and consider as most important.

The Highlights of Prescribing Information for Coumadin, the brand name of warfarin, provides health care practitioners with a half-page summary of the most commonly referred to safety information.

1. **Name of Drug.** The very first section will tell you the name of the drug. It will show you the brand name as well as the generic name, or active ingredient, in parentheses. This section also tells you what formulation it is (injection, oral, etc.) and the year the FDA approved the drug.

2. **Black Box Warning.** If there is a black box warning for the drug, it will be at the top of the page. The boxed warning provides the most important safety information about the drug. In the case of Coumadin, it warns about the risk of major or fatal bleeding.

3. **Recent Major Changes.** Below the black box warning, you will find any recent major changes to the prescribing information and the date they were made. The FDA will add or remove warnings. If you have been taking the same medication for a while, it is a good idea to check this section periodically to see if there have been new warnings added. However, this section is not always included.

4. **Indications and Usage.** This section lists all of the conditions the FDA has approved the drug to treat. Sometimes health care providers can legally prescribe drugs for off-label uses, which are uses not approved by the FDA. Such uses might not be supported by data that proves safety or effectiveness, however. All information in the prescribing information is specifically for FDA-approved uses only.

5. **Dosage and Administration.** Here you can find information about the recommended amount of the drug and how to give it to a patient. For example, the Coumadin dose depends on tests a health care provider runs, and it is specific to the patient.

6. **Dosage Forms and Strengths.** All of the different doses available from the manufacturer are listed here. Providers can recommend any dose and may increase or decrease the dose over time. Coumadin starts at 1 mg and goes up to 10 mg in its pill form, and the drug for injection comes in a vial containing 5 mg of powder. Check the label on your prescription package from the pharmacy for the dose that your provider has prescribed for you.

7. **Contraindications.** Not all medications are safe for everyone. This section tells providers who should not take the drug.

8. **Warnings and Precautions.** Warnings and precautions inform doctors about serious conditions that can occur in people taking the drug. It alerts them to health problems to watch for in their patients who take the drug. For example, people taking Coumadin might suffer rare tissue death or gangrene that may lead to amputation.

9. **Adverse Reactions.** Look here for the most common side effects suffered by people taking the drug. Coumadin's most common reactions are fatal and nonfatal bleeding. This section also provides contact information to report side effects to the manufacturer and the FDA.

10. **Drug Interactions.** Drugs listed in this section may interact with the medication, increasing or decreasing its effectiveness or causing more side effects.

11. **Use in Specific Populations.** The drug may affect people differently depending on characteristics such as age, gender, race, pregnancy or the presence of kidney or liver impairment. This section warns about safety or effectiveness concerns in these groups.

The full prescribing information expands on the information provided in the highlights section. This part of the prescribing information is the most complicated because manufacturers write it for health care providers, scientists and researchers, not patients.

The full prescribing information is written for people in the medical community and elaborates on information found in the highlights section.

In addition to the highlights, it contains information on how the drug works, how long it lasts in the body and how the body gets rid of the drug. It will also talk about animal studies, which might provide information about whether or not the drug causes cancer or infertility.

FULL PRESCRIBING INFORMATION: CONTENTS*

WARNING: BLEEDING RISK
1   INDICATIONS AND USAGE
2   DOSAGE AND ADMINISTRATION
     2.1   Individualized Dosing
     2.2   Recommended Target INR Ranges and Durations for Individual Indications
     2.3   Initial and Maintenance Dosing
     2.4   Monitoring to Achieve Optimal Anticoagulation
     2.5   Missed Dose
     2.6   Intravenous Route of Administration
     2.7   Treatment During Dentistry and Surgery
     2.8   Conversion From Other Anticoagulants
3   DOSAGE FORMS AND STRENGTHS
4   CONTRAINDICATIONS
5   WARNINGS AND PRECAUTIONS
     5.1   Hemorrhage
     5.2   Tissue Necrosis
     5.3   Systemic Atheroemboli and Cholesterol Microemboli
     5.4   Heparin-Induced Thrombocytopenia
     5.5   Use in Pregnant Women with Mechanical Heart Valves
     5.6   Females of Reproductive Potential
     5.7   Other Clinical Settings with Increased Risks
     5.8   Endogenous Factors Affecting INR
6   ADVERSE REACTIONS
7   DRUG INTERACTIONS
     7.1   CYP450 Interactions
     7.2   Drugs that Increase Bleeding Risk
     7.3   Antibiotics and Antifungals
     7.4   Botanical (Herbal) Products and Foods

8   USE IN SPECIFIC POPULATIONS
     8.1   Pregnancy
     8.3   Nursing Mothers
     8.4   Pediatric Use
     8.5   Geriatric Use
     8.6   Renal Impairment
     8.7   Hepatic Impairment
     8.8   Females of Reproductive Potential
10   OVERDOSAGE
     10.1   Signs and Symptoms
     10.2   Treatment
11   DESCRIPTION
12   CLINICAL PHARMACOLOGY
     12.1   Mechanism of Action
     12.2   Pharmacodynamics
     12.3   Pharmacokinetics
     12.5   Pharmacogenomics
13   NONCLINICAL TOXICOLOGY
     13.1   Carcinogenesis, Mutagenesis, Impairment of Fertility
14   CLINICAL STUDIES
     14.1   Atrial Fibrillation
     14.2   Mechanical and Bioprosthetic Heart Valves
     14.3   Myocardial Infarction
15   REFERENCES
16   HOW SUPPLIED/STORAGE AND HANDLING
17   PATIENT COUNSELING INFORMATION

* Sections or subsections omitted from the full prescribing information are not listed

The manufacturers also share results of clinical trials, data showing how well the drug works and its side effects from those clinical trials.

Task 1

Directions: *Match the medicine with its definition.*

(1) anaesthetic　　　A. A medicine you use for helping you to cough up mucus from your lung

(2) analgesic　　　B. A substance that prevents a poison from having bad effects

(3) antacid　　　C. A drug or gas that is given to someone before a medical operation

(4) antibiotic　　　D. A drug that reduces pain

(5) antidote　　　E. A pill that you take to help you to sleep

(6) antihistamine　　　F. A drug taken to reduce inflammation (swelling, heat, and pain)

(7) anti-inflammatory　　G. A drug used for preventing a woman from becoming pregnant

(8) contraceptive　　　H. A drug used to treat an allergy

(9) emetic　　　I. A medicine that reduces the amount of acid in your stomach

(10) expectorant　　　J. A drug that cures illnesses and infections caused by bacteria

(11) laxative　　　K. A medicine that helps you to make loose waste

(12) narcotic　　　L. A drug that makes you vomit

(1)	(2)	(3)	(4)	(5)	(6)	(7)	(8)	(9)	(10)	(11)	(12)

Task 2

Directions: *Warning information printed or placed on the bottle as stickers may vary. Explain the following sticker's meaning.*

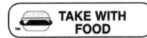

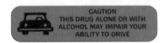

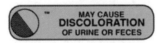

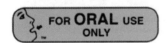

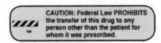

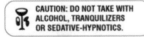

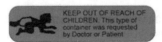

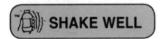

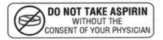

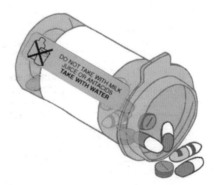

Task 3

Directions: *Find a complete English package insert of your concern and then write a pharmacy information sheet as below.*

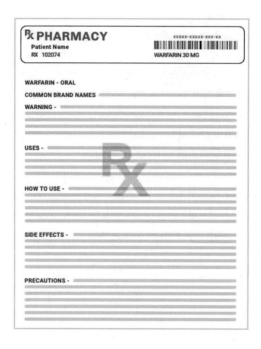

Task 4

Directions: *The label on the prescription bottle contains information from the doctor and the pharmacy about using the medication correctly. Use the guide below to identify the key sections.*

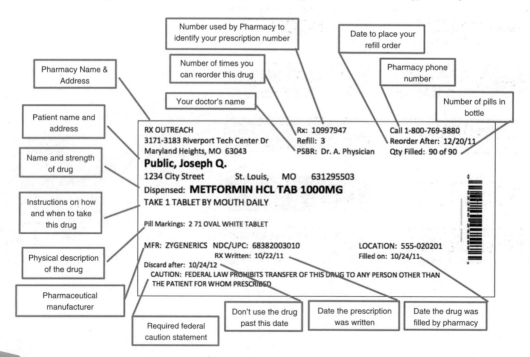

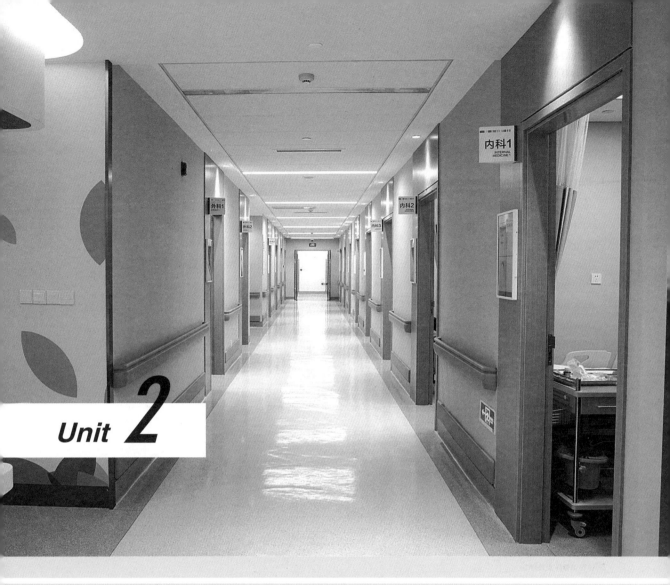

Unit 2

Disease of Human Body

√ 听力音频
√ 听力文本
√ 课件资源

Warm-up

1. Put the following diseases into one of the categories below.

cataract	stomach ulcer	pneumonia	Parkinson's disease
heart attack	glaucoma	dementia	irregular heart rhythm
diabetes	warts	gum disease	thyroid dysfunction
fracture	hysteria	kidney failure	macular degeneration
psychosis	asthma	folliculitis	contact dermatitis
cystitis	elbow tennis	cross bite	rheumatoid arthritis
gastroesophageal reflux disease (GERD)		schizophrenia	oral habits
chronic obstructive pulmonary disease (COPD)			

Musculoskeletal: _____

Hormonal: _____

Neurologic: _____

Visual: _____

Cardiovascular: _____

Lungs: _____

Skin and hair: _____

Gastrointestinal: _____

Urinary: _____

Oral and dental: _____

Psychiatric: _____

2. Discuss the category of the following symptoms with your partners.

dry mouth	anxiety	constipation	dysuria	balance problem
weight gain	fatigue	itching	heartburn	urinary incontinence
appetite loss	dry skin	hair loss	polyuria	menopause
tingling	sleep problems	sore throat	dizziness	shortness of breath

Theme Reading

Disease of Human Body

Every living thing, both plants and animals, can succumb to disease. People, for example, are often infected by tiny bacteria. Hundreds of different diseases exist. Each has its own specific diagnosis and treatment. Each is caused by its specific pathogenic microorganism. In this part, you will have an overview of the diseases of the human body.

Objectives

☆ *Understand the basic concepts about human disease.*
☆ *Describe the classifications of diseases.*
☆ *Describe the principles of diagnosis.*
☆ *List the diagnostic tests and procedures.*

A disease associated with structural changes is called an **organic** disease. In contrast, a functional disease is one in which no morphologic abnormalities can be identified even though body functions may be profoundly disturbed.

Pathology is the study of disease and a pathologist is a physician who specializes in diagnosing and classifying diseases, primarily by examining the **morphology** of cells and tissues. A clinician is any physician or other health practitioner who cares for patients.

A disease may cause various subjective manifestations, such as weakness or pain, in an affected individual: These are called symptoms. A disease may also produce objective manifestations, detectable by the clinician, which are called signs or physical findings.

A disease that causes the affected individual no discomfort or disability is called an **asymptomatic** disease or illness. The distinction between asymptomatic and symptomatic disease is one of degree, depending primarily on the extent of the disease.

The term **etiology** means cause. If the cause of a disease is known, the agent responsible is called the etiologic agent. The term **pathogenesis** refers to the manner by which a disease develops, and a pathogen is any microorganism, such as a bacterium or virus, that can cause disease.

Classifications of Disease

Diseases tend to fall into several large categories, although the diseases in a specific category are not necessarily closely related. Rather, the lesions produced by the various diseases in a category are morphologically similar or have a similar pathogenesis. Diseases are conveniently classified in the following large groups: **congenital** and **hereditary** diseases; inflammatory diseases; degenerative diseases; metabolic diseases and **neoplastic** diseases.

Congenital and Hereditary Diseases

Congenital and hereditary diseases are the result of developmental disturbances. They may be caused by genetic abnormalities, abnormalities in the numbers and distribution of chromosomes, **intrauterine** injury as a result of various agents, or interaction of genetic and environmental factors.

Inflammatory Diseases

Inflammatory diseases are those in which the body reacts to an injurious agent by means of inflammation. Some diseases in this category appear to be caused by antibodies formed against the patient's own tissues, as occurs in some uncommon diseases classified as autoimmune diseases.

Degenerative Diseases

In degenerative diseases, the primary abnormality is degeneration of various parts of the body. In some cases, this may be a manifestation of the aging process. In many cases, however, the degenerative lesions are more advanced or occur sooner than would be expected if they were age related, and they are distinctly abnormal.

Metabolic Diseases

The chief abnormality seen in metabolic diseases is a disturbance in some important metabolic process in the body.

Neoplastic Diseases

Neoplastic diseases are characterized by abnormal cell growth that leads to the formation of various types of benign and malignant tumors.

Principles of Diagnosis

The determination of the nature and cause of a patient's illness by a physician or other health practitioner is called a diagnosis. It is based on the practitioner's evaluation of the patient's subjective symptoms, the physical findings, and the results of various laboratory tests, together with other appropriate diagnostic procedures. When the practitioner has reached a diagnosis, he or she can then offer a prognosis; an opinion concerning the eventual outcome of the disease. Then, a course of treatment is instituted.

The History

The clinical history is a very important part of the evaluation. It consists of several parts: the history of the patient's current illness; the past medical history; the family history; the social history and the review of systems.

The history of the present illness **elicits** details concerning the severity, time of onset, and character of the patient's symptom. The past medical history provides details of the patient's general health and previous illnesses. The family history provides information about the health of the patient's parents and other family members. The social history deals with the patient's occupation, habits, alcohol and tobacco consumption, and similar data. The review of systems inquires as to the presence of symptoms other than discloses in the history of the present illness; such symptoms might suggest disease affecting other parts of the body.

The Physical Examination

The physical examination is a systematic examination of the patient. Any abnormalities detected on the physical examination are correlated with the clinical history. At this point, the practitioner begins to consider the various diseases or conditions that would fit with the clinical findings. Sometimes, more than one possible diagnosis needs to be considered.

Diagnostic Tests and Procedures

Diagnostic tests and procedures fall into two classifications: invasive procedures and noninvasive procedures. Invasive procedures are so-named because the patient's body is actually "invaded" in some way in order to obtain diagnostic information. Noninvasive procedures are those that entail no risk or minimal risk or discomfort to the patient. Diagnostic tests and procedures can be classified into the following major categories.

Clinical Laboratory Tests

Clinical laboratory tests can be used to determine the concentration of various constituents in the blood and urine, which are frequently altered by disease. Clinical laboratory tests are also used to evaluate the functions of organs such as clearance tests, pulmonary function tests, liver function tests, microbiologic tests and serologic tests.

Tests of Electrical Activity

Several different tests measure the electrical impulses associated with various bodily functions and activities. These include the electrocardiogram (ECG), the electroencephalogram (EEG), and the electromyogram (EMG). The most widely used of these tests is the electrocardiogram.

Radioisotope (Radionuclide) Studies

The function of various organs can be evaluated by administering a substance labeled with a radioactive material called radioisotope. One may administer a radioactive material that is filtered out or concentrated in a tissue or organ and then measure the radioactivity by radiation detectors.

Endoscopy

An **endoscopy** is an examination of the interior of the body by means of various types of rigid or flexible tubular instruments. These instruments have a system of lenses for viewing and a light source to illuminate the region being examined.

Ultrasound

Ultrasound is a technique for mapping the echoes produced by high-frequency sound waves transmitted into the body. Echoes are reflected wherever there is a change in the density of the tissue. The reflected waves are recorded on sensitive detectors, and images are produced.

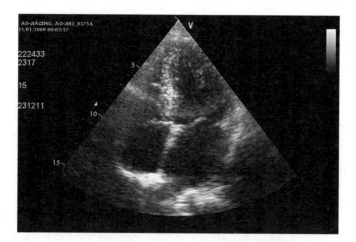

Figure 2-1 Ultrasonic picture

X-ray Examination

X-rays are passed through the part of the body to be examined, and the rays leaving the body expose an X-ray film. The extent to which the rays are absorbed by the tissues as they pass through the body depends on the density of the tissues. The X-ray image produced on the film is called radiograph or **roentgenogram**.

Abnormalities of internal organs that cannot be identified by means of standard X-ray examinations can often be discovered with computed tomographic scan (CT scan), which is performed by a highly sophisticated X-ray machine that produces images of the body in cross section.

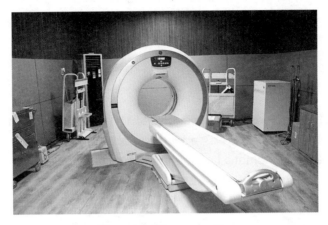

Figure 2-2 CT scan machine

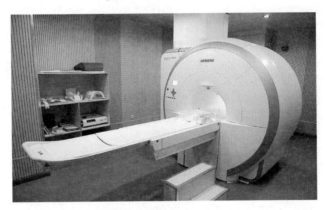

Figure 2-3 MRI machine

Magnetic Resonance Imaging

Magnetic resonance imaging (MRI) produces computer-constructed images of various organs and tissues somewhat like CT scans. MRI scans depend on the response of hydrogen **protons** contained within water molecules when they are placed in a strong magnetic field.

Positron Emission Tomography

Related to radioisotope studies but much more complex and sophisticated is one of the newest of the diagnostic imaging tests called positron emission tomography (PET), or simply

PET scans. One uses PET scans to study body functions by injecting into the subject a biochemical compound and then assessing the distribution and metabolism of the compound.

Cytologic and Histologic Examinations

Abnormal cells can often be identified in the fluids or secretions that come in contact with the epithelial surface. It is often possible to determine the cause of a patient's disease by histologic examination of a small sample of tissue removed from the affected tissue or organ. This procedure is called a **biopsy**.

Treatment

There are two different types of treatment: specific treatment and symptomatic treatment. A specific treatment is one that exerts a highly specific and favorable effect on the basic cause of the diseases. Symptomatic treatment, as the name implies, makes the patient more comfortable by alleviating symptoms but does not influence the course of the underlying disease.

Vocabulary

asymptomatic [ˌeɪsɪmptəˈmætɪk]   having no symptoms

biopsy [ˈbaɪɒpsi]   removal and pathologic examination of specimens in the form of small pieces of tissue from the living body

congenital [kənˈdʒenɪtl]   existing at or from your birth

elicit [iˈlɪsɪt]   to get information from someone by asking questions

endoscopy [enˈdɒskəpi]   procedures of applying endoscopes for disease diagnosis and treatment, which involves passing an optical instrument along either natural body pathways such as the digestive tract, or through keyhole incisions to examine the interior parts of the body

etiology [ˌiːtɪˈɒlədʒi]   cause of a disease

hereditary [hɪˈredɪtri]   able to be passed down from parent to child

intrauterine [ˌɪntrəˈjuːtərɪn]   within or situated in the uterus

morphology [mɔːˈfɒlədʒi]   the branch of biology that deals with the form and structure of organisms without consideration of function

neoplastic [ˌniːəʊˈplæstɪk]   about tumor

organic [ɔːˈgænɪk]   pertaining to the organs of human body

pathogenesis [ˌpæθəˈdʒenɪsɪs]   the mechanism by which the disease is caused; the origin and development of the disease

proton [ˈprəʊtɒn]   a very small piece of matter present in the central part of an atom

radioisotope [ˌreɪdɪəʊˈaɪsətəʊp]   a radioactive isotope

radionuclide [ˌreɪdɪəʊˈnjuːklaɪd]   a radioactive nuclide

roentgenogram [ˈrentgənəˌgræm]   an X-ray photograph

Task 1

Directions: *Select the letter of the choice that best completes the statement or answers the question.*

(1) Various subjective manifestations, such as weakness or pain, in an affected individual can be called _____.

    A. signs   B. symptoms   C. physical findings   D. diagnosis

(2) The term _____ refers to the manner by which a disease develops.

    A. pathogenesis   B. pathogen   C. pathology   D. pathologist

(3) Some degenerative lesions are _____ -related, and they are often normal.

    A. gender   B. time   C. gene   D. age

(4) Malignant tumors can be termed as _____.

    A. fibroma   B. benign tumor   C. cancer   D. sarcoma

(5) A prognosis is a prediction about the _____ of the disease.

    A. findings   B. outcome   C. treatment   D. surgery

(6) The history of the _____ illness talks about the severity, time of onset, and character of the patient's symptom.

    A. present   B. past   C. family   D. social

(7) Which of the following item is NOT related to patient's social history?

    A. Occupation.   B. Habits.

    C. Alcohol and tobacco consumption.   D. Health status of family members.

(8) _____ procedures entail no risk or minimal risk or discomfort to the patient.

    A. Noninvasive   B. Invasive   C. Diagnostic   D. Clinical

(9) Which of the following CANNOT measure the electrical activity of the body?

    A. ECG.   B. EMG.   C. MRI.   D. EEG.

(10) The extent to which the X-rays are absorbed by the tissues as they pass through the body depends on the _____ of the tissues.

    A. altitude   B. degree   C. shape   D. density

Task 2

Directions: *Label the procedures on the following pictures.*

(1)_____   (2)_____   (3)_____   (4)_____

Task 3

Directions: *Give some examples of the following terms. You may refer to the text above or search from Internet.*

Disease	Examples
(1) congenital and hereditary diseases	
(2) inflammatory diseases	
(3) degenerative diseases	
(4) metabolic diseases	
(5) neoplastic diseases	

Task 4

Directions: *Match each of the following terms in Column A with its definition in Column B.*

A	B
(1) organic	A. the branch of biology that deals with the structure of animals and plants
(2) asymptomatic	B. about tumor
(3) etiology	C. pertaining to the organs of human body
(4) biopsy	D. present at birth but not necessarily hereditary; acquired during fetal development
(5) pathogenesis	E. within or situated in the uterus
(6) neoplastic	F. cause of a disease
(7) intrauterine	G. having no symptoms
(8) endoscopy	H. the mechanism by which the disease is caused
(9) congenital	I. procedures of applying endoscopes for disease diagnosis and treatment
(10) morphology	J. removal and pathological examination of specimens in the form of small pieces of tissue from the living body

Medical Terminology

Prefixes		Terminology	Term Analysis	Definition
not, without				
a-, an-		aplasia [əˈpleɪzɪə] anemia [əˈniːmɪə]	plas=development, formation hem(o)=blood	
reverse; remove from				
de-		defibrillator [diːˈfɪbrɪleɪtə] dehydration [diːhaɪˈdreɪʃən]	fibr(o)=fiber hydr(o)=water	

(to be continued)

away from			
ab-	abductor [æb'dʌktə] abnormality [æbnɔ:'mælɪti]		
toward			
ad-, ac-, af-, ag-	adductor [ə'dʌktə] acceptor [ək'septə] afferent ['æfərənt] aggravate ['æɡrəveɪt]		
before, forward			
ante-	antenatal [ˌænti'neɪtəl] anteversion [ˌænti'vɜ:ʃən]	nat(o)=birth	
after, behind			
post-	postpartum [ˌpəʊst'pɑ:təl] postfebrile [ˌpəʊst'fi:braɪl]	part=birth feb(o)=fever	
above, beyond			
supra-	supracranial [s(j)u:prə'kreɪnɪəl] supranasal [ˌju:prə'neɪzəl]	crani(o)=skull	
below, beneath			
infra-	infracostal [ˌɪnfrə'kɑstəl] inframammary [ˌɪnfrə'mæməri]	cost(o)=rib mamm(o)=breast	
above, excessive, beyond			
hyper-	hypertension [haɪpə'tenʃn] hyperglycemia [ˌhaɪpəglaɪ'si:mɪə]	glyc(o)=sugar	
under, deficient, below			
hypo-	hypothalamus [haɪpə'θæləməs] hypothyroidism [ˌhaɪpəʊ'θaɪrɔɪdɪzəm]	thyr(o)=thyroid gland	

(to be continued)

above, over, upon			
epi-	epithelial [ˌepɪˈθiːliəl] epidermis [ˌepɪˈdɜːmɪs]	derm(o)=skin	
under, beneath			
sub-	subcutaneous [sʌbkjʊˈteɪniəs] subhepatic [ˌsʌbhɪˈpætɪk]	cut=skin hepat(o)=liver	
within			
intra-	intravenous [ˌɪntrəˈviːnəs] intramuscular [ˌɪntrəˈmʌskjələ(r)]	ven(o)=vein	
outside			
extra-	extracellular [ekstrəˈseljʊlə] extrauterine [ˌekstrəˈjuːtəraɪn]	uter(o)=uterus	
inside, within			
endo-	endocrine [ˈendəʊkrɪn; ˈendəʊkraɪn] endocarditis [ˌendəʊkɑːˈdaɪtɪs]	crin(o)=secrete cardi(o)=heart	
out			
ex-, exo-	exocrine [ˈeksəʊkraɪn; ˈeksəʊkrɪn] exotoxin [ˌeksəʊˈtɒksɪn]		
between			
inter-	intercostal [ɪntəˈkɒstəl] interneuron [ˌɪntəˈnjʊərɒn]	cost(o)=rib	
around			
circum-	circumvascular [ˌsɜːkəmˈvæskjʊlə] circumrenal [ˌsɜːkəmˈriːnəl]	vas(o)=blood vessel ren(o)=kidney	
around, surrounding			

(to be continued)

peri-	pericardial [ˌperɪˈkɑːdɪəl] periosteum [ˌperɪˈɒstɪəm]	oste(o)=bone	
up, backward, again			
ana-	anabolism [əˈnæbəlɪz(ə)m] anatomy [əˈnætəmi]	tom(o)=cut	
down, under			
cata-	catabolism [kəˈtæbəlɪzəm] catalysis [kəˈtæləsɪs]	bol(o)=throw	
against, opposite			
contra-	contrasexual [ˌkɒntrəˈsekʃʊəl] contraception [ˌkɒntrəˈsepʃən]		
against			
anti-	antibiotic [ˌæntibaɪˈɒtɪk] antiviral [ˌæntiˈvaɪrəl]	bi(o)=living thing	
abnormal, difficult, bad, impaired			
dys-	dyspepsia [dɪsˈpepsɪə] dyspnea [dɪspˈniːə]	pepsi=digestion pne(o)=breathing	
good, normal			
eu-	eugenics [juːˈdʒenɪks] eupepsia [juːˈpepsɪə]	gen(o)=production	
alongside, near, beyond, abnormal			
para-	parasympathetic [ˌpærəˌsɪmpəˈθetɪk] parathyroid [pærəˈθaɪrɔɪd]	sym=together path(o)=feeling	
through, throughout			

(to be continued)

dia-	dialysis [daɪˈæləsɪs] diagnosis [ˌdaɪəgˈnəʊsɪs]	lys(o)=separation	
two			
bi-	bisection [ˌbaɪˈsekʃən] bilateral [ˌbaɪˈlætərəl]	sect=cut later(o)=side	
half			
semi-	semicircular [semɪˈsɜːkjələ(r)] semilunar [ˌsemɪˈluːnə]		
change			
meta-	metabolism [məˈtæbəlɪzəm] metastasis [məˈtæstəsɪs]		
across			
trans-	transplantation [ˌtrænsplɑːnˈteɪʃn] transaminase [trænˈsæmɪneɪs]		
beyond, excess			
ultra-	ultrasonography [ʌltrəsəˈnɒgrəfi] ultramicroscope [ʌltrəˈmaɪkrəskəʊp]		

Vocabulary Study

Task 1

Directions: *Match each of the following terms with its definition and underline the strong part of each word where there are two or more syllables.*

(1) anemia	A. difficulty in breathing or in catching the breath
(2) dehydration	B. an abnormally large amount of sugar in the blood
(3) dyspnea	C. dryness resulting from the removal of water
(4) hyperglycemia	D. insufficient production of thyroid hormones
(5) hypothyroidism	E. a deficiency of red blood cells

(6) infracostal	A. below the liver
(7) antenatal	B. situated beneath the ribs
(8) supracranial	C. having frequencies above those of audible sound
(9) subhepatic	D. situated above, or in the roof of, the cranium
(10) ultrasonic	E. occurring or existing before birth

Task 2

Directions: *Fill in the blanks with appropriate words for body parts.*

(1) Supranasal describes the place above the _____.

(2) Intercostal means between the _____.

(3) Intracranial zone is situated within the _____.

(4) Perihepatic is the word used to describe the area surrounding the _____.

(5) Intravenous describe how the drugs are put into people's bodies through their _____.

(6) Extrauterine pregnancy occurs when a fertilized egg grows outside a woman's _____.

(7) Endocarditis refers to inflammation of the _____.

(8) Surrounding or partly surrounding the _____ is termed circumrenal.

(9) A person who has an ileectomy has had a complete or partial removal of the _____.

(10) Parathyroid refers to any one of four endocrine glands situated near the _____ gland.

Case Study 2-1

Ovarian Cancer

C.F., a 46-YO married Asian woman, works as an office manager for an insurance company. This morning, she had a follow-up visit with her oncologist and was sent to the hospital for immediate admission for possible recurrence or sequelae of her ovarian cancer. She is alert, articulate, and a reliable reporter.

CC: C.F. presents with mild, low, aching pelvic pain and low abdominal fullness. She states, "I feel like I have cramps and am bloated. Sometimes I'm so tired I cannot do my work without a short nap."

HPI: C.F. has been in remission for 14 months from aggressively treated ovarian carcinoma. She presents with mild abdominal distention and tenderness on deep palpation of the lower pelvis. C.F. claims a feeling of fullness in the lower abdomen, loss of appetite, and inability to sleep through the night. She is afraid that her cancer was not cured. Sometimes her heart races and she cannot catch her breath, but with two children in college, she cannot afford to miss work.

MEDS: Therapeutic vitamin × 1/day. Valium 5 mg every 6 hours (q6h) as needed (prn) for anxiety. Benadryl 25 mg at bedtime (hs) prn for insomnia. Echinacea tea 3 cups/day to prevent colds or flu. Ginkgo biloba 3 cups/day for energy.

ALLERGIES: NKDA, no food allergies.

PMH: C.F. was diagnosed with ovarian CA four years ago and treated with surgery, radiation, and chemotherapy. A total abdominal hysterectomy (removal of the uterus) with bilateral removal of the oviducts and ovaries was performed. At the time of surgery, the pelvic lymph nodes tested negative for disease. Chemotherapy and radiation therapy occurred after surgical recovery. C.F. has been well and capable of full ADL until four weeks ago. Childhood history is unremarkable, with normal childhood diseases, including measles, mumps, and chicken pox. C.F. was born and raised in this country. She has no other adult diseases, surgery, or injuries.

CURRENT HEALTH Hx: Denies tobacco, ETOH, or recreational drugs or substances. She exercises three to five times per week with aerobic exercise class and treadmill. She is a vegetarian and drinks one to five cups of green tea per day. Immunizations are up to date, unsure of last tetanus booster. Recent negative mammogram and negative TB test (PPD).

FAMILY Hx: Both parents alive and well. Maternal aunt died of "stomach tumor" at age 37.

Task 3

Directions: *Select the best answer to the question or the statement based on the information provided in the case of ovarian cancer.*

(1) What does an oncologist refer to?
  A. A specialist in tumor or cancer.
  C. A specialist in heart disease.
  B. A specialist in kidney disease.
  D. A specialist in inflammatory disease.

(2) What was C.F. sent to the hospital for?
  A. Headache.   B. Weakness.   C. Ovarian cancer.   D. Diarrhea.

(3) Carcinoma refers to_____.
  A. cancer   B. tumor   C. inflammation   D. infection

(4) C.F's symptoms do NOT include_____.
  A. fullness in the lower abdomen   B. loss of appetite
  C. vomiting   D. inability to sleep

(5) Medications are prescribed for_____.
  A. insomnia   B. energy   C. anxiety   D. all of the above

(6) C.F. was diagnosed with ovarian CA four years ago and treatment did NOT include _____.
  A. surgery   B. psychological therapy   C. radiation   D. chemotherapy

(7) The term hysterectomy means_____.
  A. removal of the uterus   B. removal of the breast
  C. removal of the kidney   D. removal of the liver

(8) What is the exact meaning of ADL?

A. Adulthood.   B. Activities of daily living.

C. Antigen and leukemia.   D. None of the above.

(9) Which description is NOT true about C.F.?

A. She is a smoker.   B. She exercises three to five times per week.

C. She is a vegetarian.   D. She drinks green tea every day.

(10) The patient is NOT sure about_____.

A. immunizations   B. last tetanus booster   C. mammogram   D. TB test (PPD)

Case Study 2-2

Intertrochanteric Fracture

A.R., age 88, slipped on the wet grass and fell while gardening in his back yard. His neighbor was unable to help him to a standing position and called for an ambulance. A.R. had excruciating pain in his right leg, which was externally rotated, slightly shorter than his left leg, and adducted. Preoperative radiographs showed a non-displaced right intertrochanteric fracture. Intraoperatively, Mr. R. was given spinal anesthesia and positioned on an orthopedic table with his right hip abducted and secured in traction. He had an open reduction and internal fixation with a compression screw and side plate with screws. His postoperative recovery was unremarkable, although he was at risk for deep vein thrombosis, that is, blood clots in his legs. He was discharged to a rehabilitation facility for several weeks of physical therapy and assistance with activities of daily living, such as personal hygiene, dressing, eating, ambulating, and toileting.

Task 4

Directions: *Write a word or phrase from the case study that means the same as each of the following.*

(1) extreme pain _____

(2) on or from the outside _____

(3) to move or turn around _____

(4) draw a limb towards the body _____

(5) an image produced on a specially sensitized photographic film or plate by radiation, usually by X-rays or gamma rays _____

(6) breaking of hard tissue such as bone _____

(7) during the operation _____

(8) loss of bodily sensation with or without loss of consciousness _____

(9) relating to problems affecting people's joints and spines _____

(10) to wander about or move from one place to another _____

Medical Term Extension

Medical Specialists

There are many types of health care workers. Clients generally start by seeing a general practitioner, but then they are referred to a specialist. If you work at a hospital or clinic, you will interact with a variety of specialists.

☆ A **chiropractor** helps manage back and neck pain through the use of spinal adjustments to maintain good alignment.

☆ An **orthodontist** specializes in the prevention or irregularities of the teeth.

☆ An **allergist** or **immunologist** focuses on preventing and treating allergic diseases and conditions.

☆ A **dermatologist** focuses on diseases and conditions of the skin, nails, and hair.

☆ An **ophthalmologist** specializes in eye and vision care.

☆ **Obstetrician/gynecologists** (OB/GYNs) provide preventive care and disease management for female health conditions.

☆ **Cardiologists** focus on the cardiovascular system, which includes the heart and blood vessels.

☆ **Endocrinologists** treat disorders and conditions that affect the endocrine system.

☆ **Gastroenterologists** focus on the digestive system.

☆ A **nephrologist** focuses on kidney care and conditions that affect the kidneys.

☆ **Urologists** treat conditions of the urinary tract in both males and females.

☆ **Pulmonologists** focus on the organs involved with breathing.

☆ **Otolaryngologists** are sometimes known as "ear, nose, and throat" (ENT) doctors.

☆ A **neurologist** treats conditions of the nerves, spine, and brain.

☆ A **psychiatrist** is a doctor who treats mental health conditions.

☆ **Oncologists** treat cancer and its symptoms.

☆ A **radiologist** specializes in diagnosing and treating conditions using medical imaging tests.

☆ A **rheumatologist** diagnoses and treats rheumatic diseases.

☆ **General surgeons** perform surgical procedures on many organs and bodily systems.

☆ An **orthopedic surgeon** specializes in diseases and conditions of the bones, muscles, ligaments, tendons, and joints.

☆ **Cardiac surgeons** perform heart surgery and may work with a cardiologist to determine what a person needs.

☆ **Anesthesiologists** focus on a person's well-being before, during, and after surgery. This may include administering pain medicine, relaxation medication, or medicine to put a person to sleep.

☆ A **pediatrician** is a medical doctor who specializes in the care of infants, children, and adolescents.

☆ A **geriatrician** specializes in the treatment of old age.

☆ A **pharmacist** is a person who fills prescriptions and gives medicine.

☆ An **audiologist** diagnoses and treats hearing and balance problems.

☆ **Physical therapists** are movement experts who improve quality of life through prescribed exercise, hands-on care, and patient education.

☆ A **therapist** provides treatment and rehabilitation.

Task 5

Directions: *Can you figure out the medical specialists in these pictures? Write down these medical specialists and list the main areas they specialize in.*

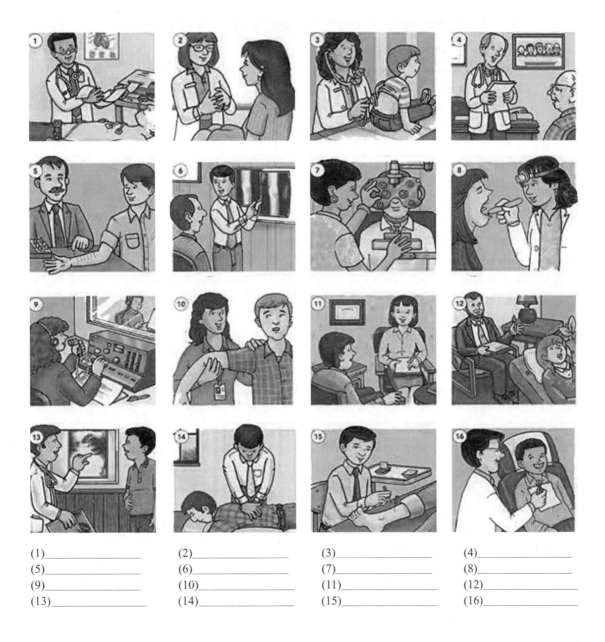

(1)_____   (2)_____   (3)_____   (4)_____
(5)_____   (6)_____   (7)_____   (8)_____
(9)_____   (10)_____   (11)_____   (12)_____
(13)_____   (14)_____   (15)_____   (16)_____

Task 6

Directions: *Name the following departments in English.*

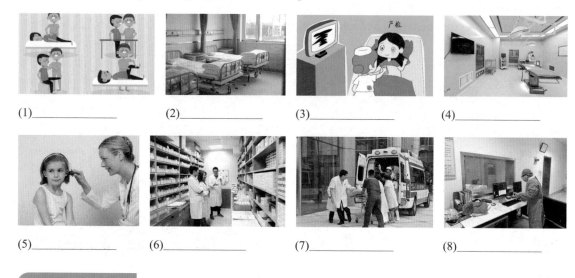

(1)_____

(2)_____

(3)_____

(4)_____

(5)_____

(6)_____

(7)_____

(8)_____

Writing

A Clinical Case Report

A case report is a description of important scientific observations that are missed or undetectable in clinical trials. This includes a rare or unusual clinical condition, a previously unreported or unrecognized disease, unusual side effects to therapy or response to treatment, and unique use of imaging modalities or diagnostic tests to assist diagnosis of a disease. Generally, a case report should be short and focussed, with its main components being the abstract, introduction, case description, and discussion.

Case reports should encompass the following five sections: an abstract, an introduction with a literature review, a description of the case report, a discussion that includes a detailed explanation of the literature review, and a brief summary of the case and a conclusion. Tables, figures, graphs, and illustrations comprise the supplementary parts and will enhance the case report's flow and clarity. Unlike original articles, case reports do not follow the usual IMRAD (introduction, methods, results, and discussion) format of manuscript organization. As the format for case reports varies greatly among different journals, it is important for authors to read carefully and follow the target journal's instructions to authors.

A case report is a detailed report of the symptoms, signs, diagnosis, treatment, and follow-up of an individual patient. It usually describes an unusual or novel occurrence and as such, remains one of the cornerstones of medical progress and provides many new ideas in medicine. It is a rapid short communication between busy clinicians who may not have time or resources to conduct large scale research. Some reports may contain an extensive review of the relevant literature on the topic.

Most journals publish case reports that deal with one or more of the following: 1) an unexpected association between diseases and symptoms; 2) an unexpected event in the course of observing or treating a patient; 3) findings that shed new light on the possible pathogenesis of a disease or an adverse effect; 4) unique or rare features of a disease; 5) unique therapeutic approaches; and 6) a positional or quantitative variation of anatomical structures from normal.

Different journals have slightly different formats for case reports. It is always a good idea to read some of the target journal's case reports to get a general idea of the sequence and format. Here is a sample of case report.

Addison's disease and its associations

Abstract

Addison's disease is a relatively rare endocrine condition resulting from adrenal insufficiency due to various causes. Weight loss is a common feature; however, patients may be seen by a variety of specialists, even requiring acute admission before the diagnosis is made. Addison's disease is commonly associated with other autoimmune diseases. In some cases such as autoimmune polyendocrine syndromes (APS) types 1 and 2, these associations are more commonly found. We present a case of one such patient who presented to the acute medical team having been referred to the gastrointestinal services in the previous year for persistent vomiting and weight loss. On review of history, the cause of vomiting and weight loss was questioned and combined with subsequent biochemical testing a diagnosis of Addison's disease was made. The patient was also noted to have other associated endocrine and autoimmune conditions.

Background

Addison's disease is not as common as other endocrine conditions such as diabetes or thyroid disease. However, it is an important consideration in acute admissions due to the associated significant morbidity and mortality. It can be very difficult to diagnose due to its varied presentation and often referrals to various specialties occur before a diagnosis is made. Many patients are only diagnosed once acutely admitted in Addison's crisis, which makes prompt diagnosis all the more important. Crisis can also be triggered by sepsis which can also mask symptoms and make the diagnosis difficult. Addison's disease is known to have associations with other conditions; therefore, knowledge of this can lead to prompt diagnosis and earlier management once this diagnosis is made.

Case presentation

A 20-year-old female patient was admitted in October with a 3-month history of persistent vomiting between 5 and 15 times a day and weight loss. She was dehydrated and unable to tolerate oral intake due to nausea and vomiting. Her bowel motions were normal; she had no problems with micturition or symptoms of infection, however had noticed significant weight loss in the preceding few months.

She had known hypothyroidism and had previously been referred directly to the gastroenterologists for persistent vomiting. She underwent an oesophagogastroduodenoscopy (OGD) which showed gastritis and therefore, she was started on proton pump inhibitor therapy. A blood test showed negative tissue transglutaminase antibodies, positive gastric parietal cell antibodies and she was scheduled for a CT enterograph.

Given this history she was treated as ongoing gastritis with vomiting secondary to the above. She had a sodium level of 133 mmol/L and low blood pressure and this was felt to be secondary to dehydration. This was treated with intravenous fluids and she was subsequently discharged on antiemetics.

The patient presented again 4 months later with persistent vomiting with some fresh blood at the end due to a Mallory-Weiss tear. She mentioned ongoing weight loss from 50 kg in August to 41 kg currently and ongoing lethargy. She described some right-sided abdominal pain and a pregnancy test was negative. She denied thyroxine abuse or forced vomiting. The patient was unsure about any relevant family history. She was a social smoker and denied any alcohol intake.

On examination she was very thin, hypotensive and tachycardic. She was clinically dehydrated and was noted to have some mild skin pigmentation.

Investigation

Her sodium levels were 129 mmol/L (normal 133–146 mmol/L), potassium levels normal at 4.9 mmol/L (3.4–5.3 mmol/L), C reactive protein (CRP) 16 (<5), haemoglobin 12.4 g/dL (12.5–16 g/dL), white cell count (WCC) 11.6 (4–11×109/L) and she had a mild eosinophilia. Given the history and findings a random cortisol was requested which came back at 2 nmol/L (102–535 nmol/L). Liver and renal function tests were normal. Thyroid stimulating hormone (TSH) was 33 mU/L (0.27–4.2 mU/L) and blood glucose was 4.5 mmol/L (4–6 mmol/L).

Differential diagnosis

On the basis of the history and investigation results, the patient was diagnosed with Addison's disease. Given her history of hypothyroidism, Addison's disease and positive gastric parietal cell antibodies; the possibility of autoimmune polyendocrine syndrome was raised.

Treatment

The patient was started on intravenous hydrocortisone 100 mg four times a day and fluids resulting in subsequent improvement.

Outcome and follow-up

A hormone profile revealed normal leutinising hormone (LH), follicle stimulating hormone (FSH), oestradiol, progesterone and prolactin with a low insulin-like growth factor (IGF). A pituitary MRI and an abdominal CT were normal with no adrenal changes.

The patient was discharged home on oral hydrocortisone and fludrocortisone tablets and educated about the importance of compliance. Unfortunately she was readmitted within the next 6 months with a further episode of Addison's crisis due to poor compliance.

Discussion

The above case highlights the importance of reviewing previous admissions and to think of other differential diagnoses especially when the presenting symptom is similar. The patient had been initially referred to the gastroenterologists; therefore, subsequent admissions were put down to a gastrointestinal cause despite there being limited improvement in symptoms. However given the ongoing weight loss despite no underlying cause on previous investigations, it was important to rule out other diagnoses and eventually the diagnosis of

Addison's disease was made almost 1 year after symptoms presented.

Addison's disease is a relatively rare condition with an annual incidence of 4 million in the western population. It can be very difficult to diagnose and easily missed due to its presentation with non-specific symptoms.

The delay in diagnosis is not uncommon and patients can be seen by various healthcare professionals including gastroenterologists or psychiatrists before being correctly diagnosed.

The wide variety in symptoms means that the diagnosis can be attributed to other conditions and the more cardinal features such as skin or mucous membrane pigmentation may be missed although these may not always be present.

Anorexia or hypotension may be relevant however are again non-specific as they be explained by alternative diagnoses such as an underlying infection.

Investigations can provide many clues to the clinician to make them suspect Addison's disease. On routine blood tests the patient may have hyponatraemia and/or hyperkalaemia, hypoglycaemia, eosinophilia. Raised TSH may be a feature and sometimes Addison's disease can be worsened by starting thyroxine.

A clinician may then suspect the diagnosis and consider a random cortisol level. However, this can be inaccurate due to the circadian rhythm of cortisol production with peak levels in the morning and low levels at midnight and also an increase in production in times of stress. An unusually low cortisol in the presence of clinical features of Addison's disease should prompt a diagnosis and this may be confirmed by a trial of hydrocortisone.

The key test for diagnosis is a short synacthen test however this can be difficult in the crisis scenario as intravenous hydrocortisone should be started immediately. Cortisol and adrenocorticotropic hormone (ACTH) levels should also be taken prior to steroid administration.

In the non-acute setting, Synacthen or synthetic ACTH (also called tetracosactrin) can be administered either intravenously or intramuscularly. A typical test involves baseline cortisol levels taken (0 min) followed by administration of 250 μg tetracosactrin and then repeat cortisol levels taken at 30 min (and 60 min in some cases). The level suggesting intact adrenal gland function has varied from between 400 and 550 nmol/L but the generally agreed level is 525 nmol/L.

About half of the patients with Addison's disease are diagnosed only after an acute adrenal crisis. It is a medical emergency often precipitated by an infection or other forms of stress in an undiagnosed or inadequately treated patient with Addison's disease. In this condition, patients present acutely unwell with severe dehydration, hypotension or circulatory shock.[4]

There are known autoimmune associations with Addison's disease. Thomas Addison described the presence of pernicious anaemia and vitiligo when describing his eponymous condition. Fifty per cent of patients with Addison's disease have an associated autoimmune disease with the most common being thyroid disease.

Addison's disease can be associated with other autoimmunity therefore if a past medical history reveals conditions such as vitiligo, thyroid disease, coeliac disease or atrophic gastritis then this raises the suspicion of another autoimmune diagnosis. The above patient had hypothyroidism and positive gastric cell antibodies. This also suggested the possibility of autoimmune polyendocrine syndrome (APS).

The Introduction gives a brief overview of the problem that the case addresses, citing relevant literature where necessary. The Introduction generally ends with a single sentence describing the patient and the basic condition that he or she is suffering from.

The Case Presentation provides the details of the case in the following order: patient description, case history, physical examination results, results of pathological tests and other investigations, treatment plan, expected outcome of the treatment plan and actual outcome. The author should ensure that all the relevant details are included and unnecessary ones excluded.

The Discussion is the most important part of the case report. It will convince the journal that the case is publication worthy. This section should start by expanding on what has been said in the Introduction, focusing on why the case is noteworthy and the problem that it addresses. This is followed by a summary of the existing literature on the topic. (If the journal specifies a separate section on literature review, it should be added before the Discussion.) This part describes the existing theories and research findings on the key issue in the patient's condition. The review should narrow down to the source of confusion or the main challenge in the case. Finally, the case report should be connected to the existing literature, mentioning the message that the case conveys. The author should explain whether this corroborates with or detracts from current beliefs about the problem and how this evidence can add value to future clinical practice.

A case report ends with a Conclusion or with summary points, depending on the journal's specified format. This section should briefly give readers the key points covered in the case report. Here, the author can give suggestions and recommendations to clinicians, teachers, or researchers. Some journals do not want a separate section for the conclusion: it can then be the concluding paragraph of the Discussion section.

Task 1

Directions: *Find more samples of case reports and identify their category.*

Samples	Category of Case Report
	An unexpected association between diseases or symptoms
	An unexpected event in the course of observing or treating a patient
	Findings that shed new light on the possible pathogenesis of a disease or an adverse effect
	Unique or rare features of a disease
	Unique therapeutic approaches
	A positional or quantitative variation of the anatomical structures

Task 2

Directions: *Structure the case report according to the general journal format.*

- Abstract/Summary
- Introduction
- Case Presentation
    - Patient's description
    - Medical history
    - Physical examination
    - Analysis of test results
    - Differential diagnosis
    - Treatment plan and outcomes
- Discussion
    - Etiology/pathophysiology
    - Literature review
    - Ethical dilemmas (if any)
- Conclusion

Task 3

Directions: *Use the patient's notes to write a textbook style of case presentation without headings.* *(Remember to anonymize the data if necessary!)*

(1) Laboratory testing. Cholesterol levels high, 300 mg/dL. Other tests negative.

_____

_____

_____

_____

(2) Name John Smith   Sex male

C/O nausea, recurrent vomiting, colicky abdominal pain, 5 days

PH hypertension

_____

_____

_____

_____

(3) PE overweight, afebril, sweaty, distress
BP 140/90 HR 110   SaO2 97%
Nerological reflexic weakness both legs, symmetrically

_____

_____

_____

_____

(4) Diagnosis gallstone ileus
Intervention enterotomy & cholelithotomy (5.2×3.6 cm)
Outcome good

_____

_____

_____

Task 4

Directions: *Complete an abstract for the case report below.*

Recurrent Gastric Metal Bezoar: A Rare Cause of Gastric Outlet Obstruction

Background

Bezoars are accumulation of foreign bodies formed of partially digested or non-digested foreign material in the gastrointestinal (GI) tract; most commonly found in the stomach but can be seen elsewhere in the digestive tube. Several types of bezoars are named according to the material from which they are composed. It could be food boluses composed of loose aggregate of food items, lactobezoar formed by inspissated milk usually seen in infants, pharmacobezoar formed by medical tablets and masses of drugs, phytobezoars composed of indigestible plant material, diospyrobezoar a type of phytobezoar formed by persimmons, trichobezoar formed by ingestion of hair and the least frequent being metal bezoar, usually seen in patients having psychiatric disorders. Few cases have been reported in the literature.

We present a case of a psychiatric man who was operated several times due to relapsing massive metal bezoars despite psychiatric treatment.

Case presentation

A 52-year-old male patient with chronic psychosis and under specific psychotic treatment, presented in May 2012 with signs and symptoms of gastric outlet obstruction due to the ingestion of metal bezoar, which was removed endoscopically. Eight months later, he was readmitted and operated because of failing endoscopic total removal of the different metals ingested. These bezoars were nails, knifes, screws, nuts, spoon handles, screwdriver head, washer, pebbles, coins and iron wire. Between 2013 and 2016, he was readmitted and operated two times in another institution for gastric metal bezoars after failed endoscopic removal in each intervention. The patient had laparotomy and metal bezoars were removed via gastrotomy.

Lately in December 2016, he was presented to the emergency department with fever and nausea; on physical examination, his vital signs were within normal limits except a moderate sinus tachycardia 110/min and 38°C. He was pale and dehydrated. Abdominal examination noted guarding throughout the abdomen, maximally in the epigastrium. A mobile mass was palpable in the left upper quadrant and epigastrium. He was admitted with provisional diagnosis of generalised peritonitis due to gastric perforation.

Blood tests revealed that the patient was septic with a haemoglobin level of 13 g/dL; peripheral white cell count was 20.1 109/L with neutrophils 85%. C-reactive protein was 200 mg/L, urea 15 mmol/L and normal creatinine. Abdominal CT scan showed a foreign body mass in the gastric region and small bowels associated with pneumoperitoneum and free intra-abdominal fluid.

Differential diagnosis includes ulcer perforation, left transverse colon tumour. The patient ultimately underwent an open laparotomy, bezoars were removed via gastrotomy and many enterotomies since the radiologic perioperative findings help us to localise all the materials and to check for their total removal to prevent recurrence. The postoperative course was uneventful and the patient was discharged on postoperative day 15 with a referral to behavioural and mental health providers.

Discussion

Bezoars are uncommon findings in the GI tract; they are composed of a wide variety of material depending on the type of the ingestion. Metal bezoar are the least common and very few cases are described in the literature. Bezoars are usually intentionally ingested, thus they occur in normal stomachs and are caused by foreign bodies that cannot bypass the pylorus. After reviewing the literature, metal bezoar was reported seven times. The first report was in 1956 by Salb and the second by Kaplan et al in 2005; later several cases were reported. None of the reported case was recurrent, complicated or massive.

However, other bezoars could occur in "abnormal" stomach, for instance, in cases of decreased gastric motility (eg, diabetes mellitus, previous vagotomy, drugs), previous gastrectomy (Billroth, gastric bypass), hypochlorydria, gastric stasis, loss of pyloric function and hypothyroidism. Clinical manifestations vary widely depending on the location of the bezoar that could be anywhere in, the digestive tract and can go from asymptomatic, non-specific symptoms to more serious intestinal obstruction, GI bleeding, perforation and peritonitis. Metal bezoar can be seen on plain radiographs unless they are radiolucent but CT scan is usually necessary and help identifying localisation and possible complications due to these foreign bodies. Gastroscopy confirms the diagnosis, defines the type of the bezoar and could treat the bezoar by its removal if they were small and technically feasible. Although different treatments have been suggested to treat phyto-tricho-bezoars such as coca-cola, papaine saline and other chemical substances for dissolution, endoscopic extraction, surgical treatment is usually necessary for metal bezoars.

Metal bezoars could be a rare cause of abdominal concern. They are generally ingested accidentally in adults, usually in infants, elderly, psychotic patients and prisoners. The patient could be asymptomatic. Surgical exploration and extraction is the treatment of choice and thorough exploration of the whole digestive tract is necessary to avoid retained materials. Psychiatric follow-up is mandatory to prevent recurrence that has been reported to be 14% in the literature.

Abstract

A 52-year-old male patient with psychiatric medical history who presented to the emergency department five times during a period of 5 years due to (1)_____ manifested mainly by (2) _____ after intentionally ingesting metals and which necessitate several surgical interventions. Lately, he presented with (3) _____ due to gastric perforation from metal bezoars. Chronic abdominal symptoms in patient having a psychiatric disorder can be due to (4) _____. Treatment is often surgical and the whole digestive tract should be explored to avoid (5) _____.

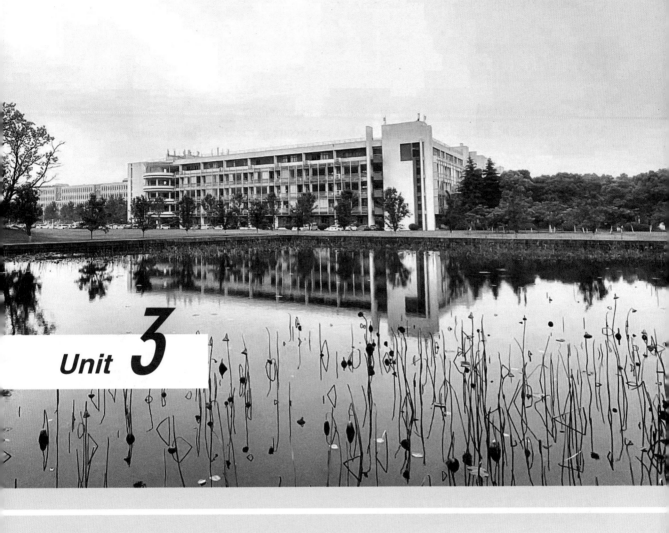

Unit *3*

The Digestive System

√ 听力音频
√ 听力文本
√ 课件资源

Warm-up

1. What kinds of digestive problems did you ever experience?
2. What are common digestive symptoms that can occur in the digestive system?

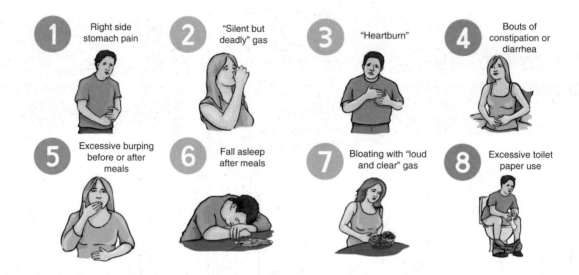

Theme Reading

The Digestive System

All food which is eaten must be changed into a soluble, absorbable form within the body before it can be used by the body. This kind of changes should be both mechanical and chemical processes, involving various organs in the digestive system. To understand them, it is necessary to trace food from the beginning of the digestive system to its end. In this part, you will have an overview of the structure and function of the digestive system.

Objectives

☆ *Describe the general function of the digestive system.*
☆ *List the structures and the functions of the digestive system.*
☆ *Describe the action of the enzymes on carbohydrates, fats and proteins.*
☆ *Trace food from the beginning of the digestive process to the end.*

Many people spend a third of their time consciously trying to control how to get food into their digestive tracts and another third thinking about how that food is doing when it gets into their digestive tracts and another third of their time consciously trying to control how to get their food **Intake** out of their digestive tracts. However, once food is swallowed, the conscious ability to control the passage of food is almost completely lost. When the food reaches the point of **elimination**, some conscious control is again reestablished in the digestive system.

The **gastrointestinal** tract or as people call it, the digestive system, has the main purpose of breaking down food, both solid and fluid into **sustenance** for the various tissues and systems in the body. A normal digestive tract squeezes the utmost benefit from what it eats. **Feces** are the products left over when the body has selected everything that is of use from the food that has been eaten.

The distance of the digestive system ranges from the mouth to the bottom of the trunk, which when we look at it, seems like no more than two or three feet, but is really about 30 feet and like a railway station consisting of signals, checkpoints and control devices in a turning, zigzagging, coiling track system.

From the moment when the three main types of food—**carbohydrates**, fats and proteins—enter the mouth, they are exposed to chemical and mechanical actions that begin to break them apart so that they can be absorbed through the intestinal walls into the circulatory system.

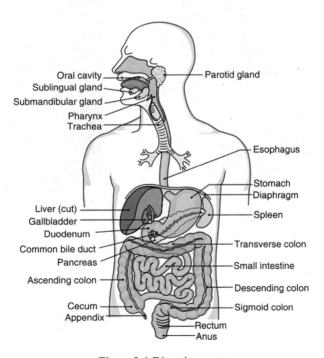

Figure 3-1 Digestive system

Chemical Digestion

Stomach

About 10 inches down the esophagus, the swallowed food or bolus is now fairly well minced and turned into a pulpy mass as it passes into the stomach. The function of the stomach is best described as a food processing unit (similar to one you may have in your kitchen) and a storage cistern. It looks like a deflated balloon when empty, but when full, it becomes about a foot long and six inches wide, able to hold about two quarts of food and drink. The stomach is both chemical and mechanical. Various chemicals in the stomach like the digestive **enzymes pepsin**, **rennin**, and **lipase** interact to break down the food. In addition, **hydrochloric acid** creates suitable environment for the enzymes and assists in the digestion. Also, watery **mucus** provides a protective lining for the muscular walls of the stomach so it will not be digested by the acid or enzymes. The mechanical action of the muscles in the stomach constrict and relax in a continuous motion blending, whipping and stirring the stomach's contents into **chyme**, a pulpy substance that can be handled by the small intestine.

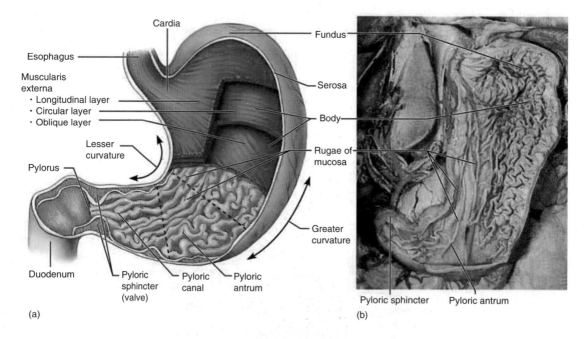

Figure 3-2 Stomach

Small Intestine

The small intestine is the longest organ of the digestive tract. It is divided up indiscriminately into three sections: the **duodenum**, the **jejunum** and the **ileum**.

Duodenum

This is the place where the ultimate destruction of food digestion reaches its completion and where the acidity of chyme is nullified. The nutrients in the food eaten many hours ago have almost been diminished to molecules small enough to be absorbed through the intestinal walls into the bloodstream. Carbohydrates are diminished into simpler sugars; proteins into amino acids; and fats into fatty acids and **glycerol**. Enzymes are secreted by the walls of the duodenum and unite with the bile (essential for the digestion and absorption of tenacious fatty materials) and pancreatic enzymes in the duodenum.

Jejunum

Peristalsis pushes the nutrient liquid out of the duodenum into the first reaches of the jejunum. A greater number of **villi**, microscopic, hair-like structures, begin to absorb amino acids, sugars, fatty acids and glycerol from the digested contents of the small intestine, and make their way to other parts of the body. This part of the small intestine executes a digestive operation so that what is passed on to the large intestine is a thin watery substance almost completely devoid of nutrients.

Ileum

This is the place which is about a third of the small intestine. The greatest number of the estimated five or six million villi in the small intestine are found along the ileum, making it the main absorption locale of the gastrointestinal tract. The villi here are always in a fretful movement: oscillating, pulsating, lengthening, shortening, and growing narrower then wider, extorting every particle of nutrient.

The Liver, Gallbladder and Pancreas

Legitimately, these three organs lie outside of the gastrointestinal tract. Nevertheless, digestive fluids from all three meet like intersections of a railway track at the common bile duct and their movement from there into the duodenum is controlled by a **sphincter** muscle. The pancreas is a producer of digestive

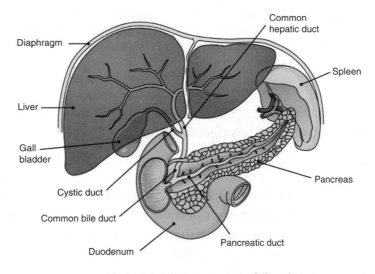

Figure 3-3 Accessory organs of digestion

enzymes. The gallbladder is a small reservoir for bile. The liver reproduces nutrients so that they can be used for cell-rebuilding and energy.

Large Intestine

There is a merger between the ileum and the **cecum**, the first section of the large intestine. Any solid substances that flow into the large intestine through the ileocecal valve (which prevents back flow into the small intestine) are as a rule indigestible or are bile constituents. What the cecum primarily inherits is water.

What the large intestine essentially does, other than act as a passageway for removal of body wastes, is to act as a provisional reservoir for water. There are no villi in the large intestine and peristalsis is much less forceful than in the small intestine. As water is absorbed, the contents of the large intestine change from a watery liquid and are compressed into semisolid feces. Nerve endings in the large intestine signal the brain that it is time for a bowel movement. The fecal material moves through the colon down to several remaining inches known as the **rectum** and out through the **anus**, an opening controlled by the outlet valves of the large intestine.

Table 3-1   Digestive Enzymes Involved in Human Digestion

Site of enzyme origin	Enzyme	Nutrient it breaks down	Product of enzyme action	Place of enzyme action
salivary glands	salivary amylase	carbohydrates-sugars	simple sugars	mouth
gastric glands	pepsin	proteins	amino acids	stomach
liver	bile	fats/lipids	emulsified fats	small intestine
small intestine	maltase, lactase, sucrase	Carbohydrates	simple sugars	small intestine
pancreas	trypsin, lipase, amylase	proteins, fats/lipids, carbohydrates	amino acids, glycerol/ fatty acids, simple sugars	small intestine

Mechanical Digestion

Mechanical digestion takes place in the mouth, where the saliva, teeth and tongue all play an important role in this digestive process.

Saliva

The smallest taste, smell and anticipation of food send signals to the brain. The brain in turn sends messages to a system of salivary glands. **Saliva** is essentially made up of water and begins to soften up the food so it can pass more smoothly down the throat. Besides water, there is also a very special substance, an enzyme called **ptyalin**, whose main task is to break down the food into simpler forms.

Teeth

The aftermath of the action of the teeth in digestion results in two outcomes: havoc and devastation. The teeth are gears to demolish chunks of food by a series of actions such as clamping, slashing, piercing, grinding and crushing. The teeth do the first drastic destruction to food in the digestive system.

Tongue

The tongue consists of four types of taste buds—salty, sweet, sour and bitter—and is a very maneuverable and pliable

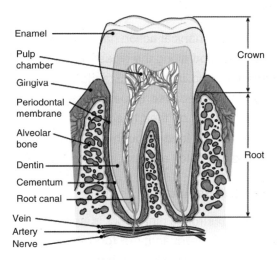

Figure 3-4 A molar tooth

arrangement of muscle. It helps to remove and dislocate food particles in the teeth and shifts food around in the mouth in order to assist with the all important act of swallowing. The act of swallowing food, which at this place in the system is called a **bolus**, brings many organs into action. As the top of your tongue presses up against the hard **palate**, the roof of your mouth, food is shoved to the back of the mouth. This action in turn brings the soft palate and **uvula** (the place at the very back of the mouth where there is a teardrop shape located) into action. They keep the food from being misguided toward the nose. Once past the soft palate, the food is in the **pharynx**, a train station with two tracks, one leading to the **trachea** (windpipe), the other to the esophagus (food pipe). The epiglottis projects out from the trachea side and helps to admit free movement of air as it is swallowed and at the same time restricts entrance to the esophagus. The larynx provides the **epiglottis** with most of its muscle for movement. It applies an upward force that helps to relax some tension on the esophagus, so that food enters where it is meant to go, down the esophagus and not down the windpipe. Many people have experienced at some time or another when the swallowing action did not go as it was supposed to.

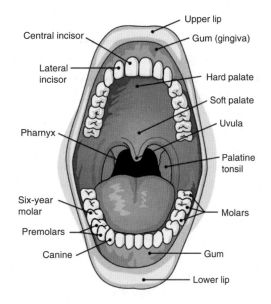

Figure 3-5 The mouth

Peristalsis

This mechanical action has to do with sets of muscles that cooperate to move both liquid and solid food along the digestive tract. In other word, it pushes food along your esophagus, stomach, and intestine. Gravitational pull is lessened in a sense when food enters the esophagus because of peristalsis. Peristalsis helps a person to swallow lying down or even standing on their head. Peristalsis has another essential task besides assisting in the movement of food through the body. It also helps to knead, agitate and pound the solid residue that is left after the teeth or those without teeth, the gums, have done their best.

Digestive Sphincters

The gastrointestinal tract is supplied with a number of muscular valves. These control and direct the quantity of food that goes through the digestive tract and inhibit the back movement of partially digested food.

Vocabulary

anus [ˈeɪnəs]   excretory opening at the end of the alimentary canal

bolus [ˈbəʊləs]   a small round soft mass (as of chewed food)

carbohydrate [ˈkɑːbəʊˈhaɪdreɪt]   an essential structural component of living cells and source of energy for animals, including simple sugars with small molecules as well as macromolecular substances

cecum [ˈsiːkəm]   the first section of your large intestine that is shaped like a bag and is open at one end

chyme [kaɪm]   a semiliquid mass of partially digested food that passes from the stomach through the pyloric sphincter into the duodenum

digestive [daɪˈdʒestɪv]   relating to or having the power to cause or promote digestion

duodenum [ˌdjuːəˈdiːnəm]   the first section of the small intestine, just below the stomach

elimination [ɪˌlɪmɪˈneɪʃən]   the process of getting rid of something that is not wanted or needed

enzyme [ˈenzaɪm]   any of several complex proteins that are produced by cells and act as catalysts（催化剂）in specific biochemical reactions

epiglottis [ˌepɪˈglɒtɪs]   a flap of cartilage that covers the windpipe while swallowing

feces [ˈfiːsiːz]   solid excretory product evacuated from the bowels

gastrointestinal [ˌgæstrəʊɪnˈtestɪnəl]   relating to the stomach and the intestines

glycerol [ˈglɪsərɒl]   a sweet syrupy trihydroxy alcohol obtained by saponification of fats and oils

hydrochloric acid [ˌhaɪdrəˈklɒrɪk] [ˈæsɪd]   a colourless, strong acid containing hydrogen and chlorine

ileum [ˈɪlɪəm]   the part of the small intestine between the jejunum and the cecum

intake [ˈɪnˌteɪk]   the amount of something that you eat or drink

jejunum [dʒɪˈdʒuːnəm]   the part of the small intestine between the duodenum and the ileum

lipase [ˈlɪpeɪs]   an enzyme secreted in the digestive tract that catalyze the breakdown of fats into individual fatty acids that can be absorbed into the bloodstream

mucus [ˈmjuːkəs]   protective secretion of the mucous membranes; in the gut it lubricates the passage of food and protects the epithelial cells; in the nose, throat and lungs, it can make it difficult for bacteria to penetrate

the body through the epithelium
palate [ˈpælət]　the upper surface of the mouth that separates the oral and nasal cavities
pepsin [ˈpepsɪn]　an enzyme produced in the stomach that splits proteins into peptones
peristalsis [ˌperɪˈstælsɪs]　the process of wave like muscle contractions of the alimentary tract that moves food along
pharynx [ˈfærɪŋks]　the part of your throat that leads from your mouth to your esophagus
ptyalin [ˈtaɪəlɪn]　an amylase secreted in saliva
rectum [ˈrektəm]　the terminal section of the alimentary canal from the sigmoid flexure to the anus
rennin [ˈrenɪn]　an enzyme that occurs in gastric juice, causing milk to coagulate
saliva [səˈlaɪvə]　a clear liquid secreted into the mouth by the salivary glands and mucous glands of the mouth, moistening the mouth and starts the digestion of starches
sphincter [ˈsfɪŋktə]　a ring of muscle that contracts to close an opening
sustenance [ˈsʌstənəns]　the act of sustaining life by food or providing a means of subsistence
tenacious [tɪˈneɪʃəs]　continue for a long time and are difficult to change
trachea [trəˈkiːə]　membranous tube with cartilaginous rings that conveys inhaled air from the larynx to the bronchi
uvula [ˈjuːvjələ]　a small pendant fleshy lobe at the back of the soft palate
villus [ˈvɪləs]　a minute hairlike projection on mucous membrane

Task 1

Directions: *Select the letter of the choice that best completes the statement or answers the question.*

(1) The gastrointestinal tract includes the mouth, _____ , esophagus, stomach, small intestine, and large intestine.
　A. liver　　　　B. larynx　　　　C. pancreas　　　　D. pharynx

(2) The accessory organs of the alimentary canal are the tongue, teeth, salivary glands, pancreas, liver and _____.
　A. stomach　　　B. esophagus　　　C. gallbladder　　　D. colon

(3) The involuntary muscle action of alimentary canal is called _____.
　A. pushing　　　B. peristalsis　　　C. stenosis　　　D. contraction

(4) Semiliquid food entering the small intestine is called _____.
　A. chyle　　　B. ptyalin　　　C. chyme　　　D. bolus

(5) Amylase allows us to digest_____.
　A. carbohydrates　　B. proteins　　　C. fats　　　D. all of these

(6) Food is absorbed in the small intestine through the _____.
　A. villi　　　B. submucosa　　　C. peritoneal lining　　　D. mucus

(7) The last portion of the small intestine is the _____.
　A. cecum　　　B. duodenum　　　C. ileum　　　D. jejunum

(8) What is produced by the liver and helps the body absorb fats?

A. Bolus.   B. Appendix.   C. Bile.   D. Colon.

(9) Which of the following is NOT part of the large intestine?

     A. Cecum.   B. Appendix.   C. Ileum.   D. Sigmoid colon.

(10) The pharynx connects the nasal and oral cavities to the _____. It serves both the respiratory and digestive systems as a channel for air and food.

     A. larynx only   B. esophagus only

     C. larynx and esophagus   D. uvula

Task 2

Directions: *Label the organs of the digestive system.*

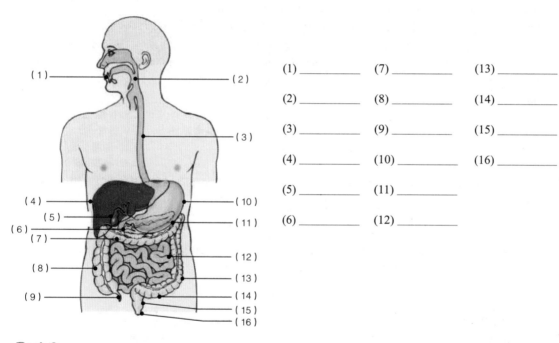

(1) _____   (7) _____   (13) _____

(2) _____   (8) _____   (14) _____

(3) _____   (9) _____   (15) _____

(4) _____   (10) _____   (16) _____

(5) _____   (11) _____

(6) _____   (12) _____

Task 3

Directions: *Fill in the following table based on the text above or relevant information from the Internet and then talk about the digestive process.*

Structure	Function
(1) mouth	
(2) esophagus	
(3) stomach	
(4) duodenum	
(5) appendix	
(6) gallbladder	
(7) liver	

(to be continued)

(8) pancreas	
(9) colon	
(10) rectum	

Task 4

Directions: *Match each of the following terms in Column A with its definition in Column B.*

A	B
(1) chyme	A. the terminal portion of the small intestine
(2) saliva	B. the fleshy mass that hangs from the soft palate, aiding in speech production
(3) anus	C. the semiliquid partially digested food that moves from the stomach into the small intestine
(4) villi	D. wave-like contractions of an organ's walls, moving material through an organ or a duct
(5) feces	E. the distal opening of the digestive tract
(6) uvula	F. an appendage; the narrow tube of lymphatic tissue attached to the cecum; the vermiform appendix
(7) appendix	G. the clear secretion released into the mouth that moistens food and contains a starch-digesting enzyme
(8) peristalsis	H. organic catalyst
(9) ileum	I. tiny projections in the lining of the small intestine that absorb digested foods into the circulation
(10) enzyme	J. the waste material eliminated form the intestine; stool

Medical Terminology

Roots	Terminology	Term Analysis	Definition
cheek / bucca			
bucc(o) ['bʌkəʊ]	bucca ['bʌkə] extrabuccal [ekstrə'bʌkəl]		
mouth / oral cavity			
or(o) ['ɔːrəʊ]	peroral [pə'ɔːrəl] oropharyngeal [ˌɔːrəˌfærɪn'dʒiːəl]	-al=pertaining to	
stom(o) ['stəʊməʊ] stomat(o) ['stəʊmətəʊ]	stomatitis [ˌstəʊmə'taɪtɪs] stomatomycosis [ˌstəʊmətəʊmaɪ'kəʊsɪs] peristomatous [ˌperɪ'stəʊmətəs]	myc(o)=fungus	

(to be continued)

lip			
labi(o) [ˈleɪbɪəʊ]	interlabial [ˌɪntɜˈleɪbɪəl] labiodental [ˌleɪbɪəʊˈdentl]		
cheil(o) [ˈkaɪləʊ]	cheiloplasty [ˈkaɪləplæsti] cheilognathopalatoschisis [ˌkaɪləʊˌneɪθəʊˌpælɑˈtɒskɪsɪs]	gnath(o)=jaw	
tongue			
lingu(o) [ˈlɪŋgwəʊ]	sublingual [sʌbˈlɪŋgwəl] linguodental [lɪŋgwəʊˈdentəl]	sub-=under	
gloss(o) [ˈglɒsəʊ]	glossotomy [glɒˈsɒtəmɪ] glossopharyngeal [ˌglɒsəʊˌfærɪnˈdʒɪːəl]		
teeth			
odont(o) [ɒˈdɒntəʊ]	orthodontia [ˌɔːθəʊˈdɒnʃɪə] periodontal [ˌperɪɒˈdɒntl]	orth(o)=straight	
dent(o) [ˈdentəʊ]	dentalgia [denˈtældʒɪə] dentin [ˈdentɪn]		
gums / gingiva			
gingiv(o) [ˈdʒɪndʒɪvəʊ]	gingivitis [ˌdʒɪndʒɪˈvaɪtɪs] gingivectomy [dʒɪndʒɪˈvektəmɪ]		
drool / saliva			
saliv(o) [sælɪvəʊ]	salivary [ˈsælɪvəri] hypersalivation [ˌhaɪpəˌsælɪˈveɪʃən]	-ary=pertaining to	
sial(o) [ˈsaɪələʊ]	sialorrhea [saɪələʊˈriːə] sialoangiitis [ˌsaɪələʊˌændʒɪˈaɪtɪs]		
palate			

(to be continued)

palat(o)	palatine		
['pælətəʊ]	['pælətaɪn]		
	palatoplasty		
	['pælətə‚plæstɪ]		
uvula			
uvul(o)	uvulitis		
[ju:vjʊləʊ]	[‚ju:vjʊ'laɪtɪs]		
	uvuloptosis		
	[ju:vjʊləʊp'təʊsɪs]		
throat / pharynx			
pharyng(o)	pharyngitis		
['færɪngəʊ;	[‚færɪn'dʒaɪtɪs]		
fə'rɪngəʊ]	pharyngoxerosis	xer(o)=dryness	
pharynge	[fə‚rɪngəʊzɪə'rəʊsɪs]		
['færɪndʒɪ;	pharyngeal		
fə'rɪndʒɪ]	[fə'rɪndʒɪəl; ‚færɪn'dʒɪəl]		
tonsil			
tonsill(o)	tonsillitis		
['tɒnsɪləʊ]	[‚tɒnsɪ'laɪtɪs]		
	tonsillotome		
	[tɒn'sɪləʊtəʊm]		
esophagus / gullet			
esophag(o)	esophagogastrostomy		
[i:'sɒfəgəʊ]	[ɪ‚sɒfəgəʊgæs'trɒstəmi]		
	tracheoesophageal		
	[treɪkɪəʊɪ‚sɒfə'dʒi:əl]		
stomach			
gastr(o)	gastroenteritis		
['gæstrəʊ]	[‚gæstrəʊentə'raɪtɪs]		
	gastrorrhagia		
	[gæstrəʊ'reɪdʒɪə]		
pylorus			
pylor(o)	pylorostenosis		
[paɪ'lɒrəʊ]	[paɪ‚lɒrəstɪ'nəʊsɪs]		
	pyloroplasty		
	[paɪ'lɔ:rəplæstɪ]		
intestine, gut, bowel			
enter(o)	enteroanastomosis		
['entərəʊ]	[‚entərəʊə‚næstə'məʊsɪs]		
	enterotoxin		
	[entərəʊ'tɒksɪn]		

(to be continued)

duodenum			
duoden(o) [djuːəʊˈdiːnəʊ]	duodenoscopy [ˌdjuːəʊdɪˈnɒskəpi] duodenectomy [ˌdjuːəʊdɪˈnektəmi]	-scopy=visual examination	
jejunum			
jejun(o) [dʒɪˈdʒuːnəʊ]	jejunal [dʒəˈdʒuːnəl] jejunoileitis [dʒə,dʒuːnəʊˌɪliˈaɪtɪs] jejunorrhaphy [ˌdʒiːdʒuːˈnɒrəfi]	-rrhaphy=suture	
ileum			
ile(o) [ˈɪlɪəʊ]	ileocolitis [ˌɪlɪəʊkəˈlaɪtɪs] ileosigmoidostomy [ˌɪlɪəʊˌsɪgmɔɪˈdɒstəmi]	-itis=inflammation	
colon			
sigmoid(o) [sɪgˈmɔɪdəʊ]	perisigmoiditis [ˌperɪˌsɪgmɔɪˈdaɪtɪs] sigmoidotomy [ˌsɪgmɔɪˈdɒtəmi]	-tomy=incision	
col(o) [ˈkəʊləʊ]	colonoscope [kəʊˈlɒnəˌskəʊp] colostomy [kəˈlɒstəmi]		
cecum			
cec(o) [ˈsiːkəʊ]	cecorrhaphy [sɪˈkɔːrəfi] cecocolopexy [ˌsiːkəʊˈkəʊləˌpeksi]		
rectum			
proct(o) [ˈprɒktəʊ]	proctology [prɒkˈtɒlədʒi] proctopexy [prɒktəʊˌpeksi]	-logy=study of	
rect(o) [ˈrektəʊ]	rectovesical [ˌrektəʊˈvesɪkəl] pararectal [ˌpærəˈrektəl]		
anus			

(to be continued)

an(o) [ˈeɪnəʊ]	anoplasty [ˈeɪnəʊˌplæsti] anoscope [ˈeɪnəskəʊp]	-scope=instrument for viewing	
appendix			
append(o) [əˈpendəʊ]	appendectomy [ˌæpenˈdektəmi] appendicitis [əˌpendɪˈsaɪtɪs]		
pancreas			
pancreat(o) [ˈpæŋkrɪətəʊ] pancre(o) [ˈpæŋkrɪəʊ]	pancreatopathy [ˌpæŋkrɪəˈtɒpəθi] pancreatitis [ˌpæŋkrɪəˈtaɪtɪs] pancreatic [ˌpæŋkrɪˈætɪk] pancreolysis [pæŋkrɪˈɒlɪsɪs]	-pathy= disease of -lysis=destruction of	
liver			
hepat(o) [ˈhepətəʊ]	hepatatrophia [ˌhepətəˈtrəʊfɪə] hepatomegaly [ˌhepətəʊˈmegəli] hepatonecrosis [ˌhepətəʊneˈkrəʊsɪs]	megal(o)=enlargement	
bile			
bil(i) [ˈbɪli]	bilirubin [ˌbɪlɪˈruːbɪn] urobilinemia [ˌjʊərəʊˌbɪlɪˈniːmɪə]	rub(e)=red	
chol(e) [ˈkəʊli] chol(o) [ˈkəʊləʊ]	cholelithiasis [ˌkəʊlɪlɪˈθaɪəsɪs] cholestasis [ˌkɒlɪˈsteɪsɪs] cholecystitis [ˌkəʊlɪsɪsˈtaɪtɪs] cholelithotripsy [ˌkəʊlɪˈlɪθətrɪpsi]	-iasis=diseased condition -tripsy=crushing	
peritoneum			
peritone(o) [ˌperiˈtəʊnɪəʊ]	peritonealgia [periˌtəʊnɪˈældʒɪə] peritoneocentesis [ˌperiˌtəʊnɪəʊsenˈtiːsɪs] peritoneography [ˌperɪtəʊnɪˈɒɡrəfi]	cent-=puncture	

(to be continued)

abdomen			
lapar(o) ['læpərəʊ]	laparocele ['læpərəʊsi:l] laparoscopy [ˌlæpə'rɒskəpi]		
abdomin(o) [æb'dɒmɪnəʊ]	abdominouterotomy [æbˌdɒmɪnəʊˌju:tə'rɒtəmi] transabdominal [ˌtrænsæb'dɒmɪnəl]	uter(o)=womb	
food			
aliment(o) [æli'mentəʊ]	alimentary [æli'mentəri] hyperalimentation [ˌhaɪpəˌrælɪmən'teɪʃən]		
sit(o) ['saɪtəʊ]	parasite ['pærəsaɪt] parasitology [ˌpærəsaɪ'tɒlədʒi]		
carbon			
carb(o) ['ka:bəʊ] carbon(o) ['ka:bəʊnəʊ]	carbohydrate [ˌka:bəʊ'haɪdreɪt] hydrocarbon [ˌhaɪdrəʊ'ka:bən] carbonate ['ka:bəneɪt]	hydr(o)=water hydr(o)=hydrogen	
digestion			
peps(o) ['pepsi] pept(o)	pepsin ['pepsɪn] dyspepsia [dis'pepsiə] transpeptidase [træns'peptɪdeɪs]		
gest(o) [dʒestəʊ]	digestion [daɪ'dʒestʃən] postdigestive [ˌpəʊstdaɪ'dʒestɪv]		
stone/calculus			
lith(o) ['lɪθəʊ]	lithodialysis [ˌlɪθəʊdaɪ'ælɪsɪs] cholelithiasis [ˌkəʊlɪlɪ'θaɪəsɪs]		

Vocabulary Study

Task 1

Directions: *Match each of the following terms with its definition and underline the strong part of each word where there are two or more syllables.*

(1) sublingual	A. surgical creation of a passage between the esophagus and the stomach
(2) gingival	B. situated beneath the tongue
(3) colostomy	C. pain in the peritoneum
(4) esophagogastrostomy	D. pertaining to the gum
(5) peritonealgia	E. surgical creation of an opening into the colon

(6) appendectomy	A. crushing of a biliary calculus
(7) cholelithotripsy	B. within the liver
(8) palatoplasty	C. surgical creation of an opening into the jejunum
(9) jejunostomy	D. surgical repair of the palate
(10) intrahepatic	E. surgical removal of the appendix

Task 2

Directions: *Fill in the blanks with appropriate words for body parts.*

(1) A person with dentalgia has a pain in the _____.

(2) Someone who has gingivitis has inflammation of the _____.

(3) Labiodental sound requires the involvement of the _____ and _____.

(4) A person with gastroenteritis has inflammation of the _____ and _____.

(5) A duodenal ulcer is located in the _____.

(6) A jejunectomy is an excision of part or all of the _____.

(7) A proctoscopy is an examination of the _____.

(8) A person who has hepatitis has an inflammation of the _____.

(9) When a cholecystectomy is performed, the _____ is removed (or excised).

(10) A person who has an ileectomy has had a complete or partial removal of the _____.

(11) During a laparotomy, an incision is made into the _____.

(12) A colotomy is an incision into the _____.

(13) Enteroptosis means an abnormal descent of the _____ in the abdominal cavity.

(14) Glossoplegia is a paralysis of the _____.

(15) A person who has pylorostenosis has a constriction of the _____.

Task 3

Directions: Write a word for each of the following definitions using the word parts provided.

-al	-itis	-rrhaphy	ile(o)	-pexy
-cele	lapar(o)	col(o)	proct(o)	cec(o)

(1) suture of the cecum _____

(2) pertaining to the ileum and cecum _____

(3) hernia of the abdomen _____

(4) inflammation of the colon _____

(5) fixation of the rectum _____

sial(o)	-ist	-rrhea	-plasty	cheil(o)	-al
an(o)	orth(o)	odont(o)	peri-	pylor(o)	

(6) surgical repairing of the lip _____

(7) a dentist who corrects the position of people's teeth _____

(8) excessive production of saliva _____

(9) surrounding the anus _____

(10) surgical reshaping of opening at the base of stomach _____

-itis	-ostomy	-ectomy	-lysis	-centesis
pancreat(o)	gastr(o)	duoden(o)	peritone(o)	esophag(o)

(11) destruction of the pancreas _____

(12) surgical communication between the stomach and food pipe _____

(13) surgical puncture into the peritoneum _____

(14) inflammation of the first part of intestine _____

(15) surgical removal of the stomach _____

Case Study 3-1

Cholecystitis

G.L., a 42-year-old obese Caucasian woman, entered the hospital with nausea and vomiting, flatulence and eructation, a fever of 100.5°F, and continuous right upper quadrant (RUQ) and subscapular pain. There was no relevant past medical history or family history. Examination on admission showed rebound tenderness in the RUQ with a positive Murphy sign. Her skin, nails, and conjunctivae were yellowish, and she complained of frequent clay-colored stools. Her leukocyte count was 16,000. An ERCP and ultrasound of the abdomen suggested many small stones in her gallbladder and possibly the common bile duct. Her diagnosis was cholecystitis with cholelithiasis.

The presence of stones in the gallbladder or bile duct is referred to as cholelithiasis. The major risk factors for the development of gallstones are widely known as the "four Fs": forty, female, fat, and fair. Gallbladder stones typically have cholesterol as their main component, while bile duct stones typically consist mostly of bilirubin. Cholelithiasis is often asymptomatic, but is sometimes detected due to biliary colic or cholecystitis. When a stone becomes stuck in the common bile duct, obstructive jaundice occurs.

A laparoscopic cholecystectomy was attempted with an intraoperative cholangiogram and common bile duct exploration. Because of G.L.'s size and some unexpected bleeding, visualization was difficult, and the procedure was converted to an open approach. Small stones and granular sludge were irrigated from her common duct, and the gallbladder was removed. She had a T-tube inserted into the duct for bile drainage; this tube was removed on the second postoperative day. An NG tube in place before and during the surgery was also removed on Day 2. She was discharged on the fifth postoperative day with a prescription for prn pain medication.

Task 4

Directions: *Select the best answer to the question or the statement based on the information provided in the case of cholecystitis.*

(1) Which of the following could NOT be what the patient G.L. complained of?

　　A. I am bloated.　　　　　　　　B. I have thrown up.

　　C. I have a tenderness.　　　　　D. I feel sick.

(2) The term "flatulence" refers to _____.

　　A. the back flow of chyme

　　B. the excessive sweating during sleep

　　C. the excessive gas or air in the intestine

　　D. the contents of the stomach through the mouth

(3) The term "eructation" means _____.

　　A. frequent bowel movement

　　B. muscular motion of the gastrointestinal tract

    C. elimination of waste material through anus

    D. passing gas from the stomach through the mouth noisily

(4) Subscapular pain is located _____.

    A. near the neck   B. above the belly

    C. under the shoulder blade   D. between the ribs

(5) The physical examination of the patient showed the tenderness in the _____ of the abdomen.

    A. left upper quadrant   B. right upper quadrant

    C. right lower quadrant   D. left lower quadrant

(6) Clay-colored stools are an indication of _____.

    A. too much fat in the diet   B. fat malabsorption

    C. intestinal bleeding   D. cirrhosis

(7) The Murphy sign is positive in patients with _____.

    A. cholecystitis   B. jaundice   C. ascites   D. peptic ulcer

(8) Cholelithiasis refers to _____.

    A. the presence of stones in the gallbladder

    B. poor or painful digestion

    C. loss of appetite

    D. an ulcer in a mucous membrane

(9) Which of the following people are the high risk population for development of gallstones?

    A. Young children.   B. Senior citizen.   C. Obese women.   D. Middle-aged men.

(10) The stones formed in the gallbladder are made up of _____.

    A. amino acid   B. cholesterol   C. glycerol   D. bilirubin

Case Study 3-2

Colonoscopy

The patient is a 73-year-old female who underwent colonoscopy and polypectomy on June 10, 2007. Biopsy revealed an invasive carcinoma, and on June 12, 2007, she underwent a low anterior resection and coloproctostomy. Fourteen months later, on August 2, 2008, she was seen in the office for flexible sigmoidoscopy, and a polyp was detected. Colonoscopy was scheduled.

Description of Procedure. The fiberoptic colonoscope was introduced, and I could pass it to about 15 cm, at which point there appeared to be an anastomosis. The colonoscope passed easily through a wide-open anastomosis to 30 cm, at which point a very friable polyp, irregular, on a short little stalk, was encountered. This was snared, the coagulating current was applied, and the pedicle was severed and recovered and sent to pathology for histological identification. The colonoscope was then reintroduced and passed through the rectum to the sigmoid colon. Again the anastomosis was seen, and proximal to this, the fulgurated base of the removed polyp could be seen. No bleeding was encountered, and I continued to advance the colonoscope through the descending colon. I proceeded to advance the colonoscope through the splenic flexure in the transverse colon. Despite vigorous mechanical bowel preparation and the shortened colon from the previous resection, she had a considerable amount of stool, and it became progressively more difficult to visualize as I approached the hepatic flexure. Finally, at the hepatic flexure, I abandoned further evaluation and began to withdraw the colonoscope. The colonoscope passed through the transverse colon, splenic flexure, descending colon, sigmoid colon, rectum, and anus and was withdrawn. She tolerated the procedure well, but had some nausea. I will await the results of pathology, and in the event that it is not an invasive carcinoma, I would recommend a repeated colonoscopy in 6 months, at which time we will use a 48-hour, more vigorous mechanical bowel preparation.

Task 5

Directions: *Write a word or phrase from the case study that means the same as each of the following.*

(1) a surgical operation to remove a polyp _____

(2) referring to cancer which tends to spread throughout the body _____

(3) a connection between two normally distinct structures _____

(4) easily crumbled or broken _____

(5) blood clotting _____

(6) stalk of the polyp _____

(7) destroyed by high-frequency electric current _____

(8) a bend in the colon where the transverse colon joins the descending colon _____

(9) the process of removing feces from the colon prior to a medical or surgical procedure _____

(10) a bend in the colon, where the ascending and transverse colons join _____

Medical Term Extension

Oral Hygiene

Good oral health helps you enjoy life. It lets you: speak clearly; taste, chew, and swallow delicious and nutritious foods; and show your feelings through facial expressions such as smiling.

If you protect your oral health with good oral hygiene practices (brushing and flossing), the odds are in your favor you can keep your teeth for a lifetime.

Brushing tips:

☆ Use fluoride toothpaste. Fluoride is what protects teeth from tooth decay (cavities). It prevents decay by strengthening the tooth's hard outer surface, called enamel.

☆ Angle the bristles toward the gumline, so they clean between the gums and teeth.

☆ Brush gently using small, circular motions. Do not scrub hard back and forth.

☆ Brush all sides of each tooth.

☆ Brush your tongue.

Flossing tips:

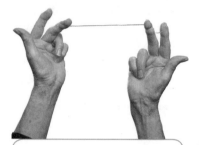 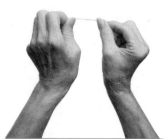 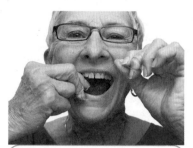

Use a string of floss about two feet long. Wrap it around the middle finger of each hand.

Grip the floss between the thumb and index finger of each hand.

Ease the floss gently between the teeth until it reaches the gumline (don't force the floss into place — this could harm the gums). Curve the floss like the letter "C" around the side of each tooth. Slide the floss up and down under the gum.

Task 6

Directions: *Name the following items in English.*

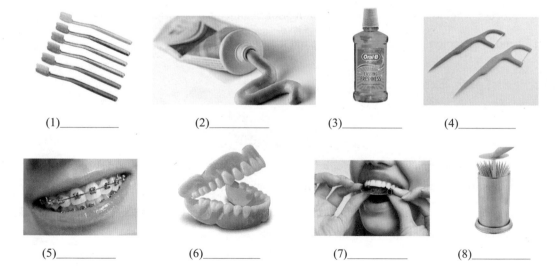

(1)_____   (2)_____   (3)_____   (4)_____

(5)_____   (6)_____   (7)_____   (8)_____

Task 7

Directions: *Complete the following quiz to test your basic knowledge on oral hygiene.*

(1) When is the best time of day to floss?

　　A. Morning.　　　B. Mid day.　　　C. Night.

(2) What is the main purpose of flossing?

　　A. To remove food from between teeth.

　　B. To loosen plaque on the sides of teeth.

　　C. To substitute for brushing.

(3) Is fluoride beneficial to your teeth?

　　A. Yes.　　　　　B. No.

(4) When flossing, how should you wrap the floss around the side of your tooth?

　　A. In a C shape.

　　B. You should not wrap it.

　　C. Diagonally, angled towards the back of your tooth.

(5) Realistically, how many times a day should you brush?

　　A. 2.　　　　　　B. 3.　　　　　　C. 4.　　　　　　D. 5.

(6) How long should you brush your teeth for?

　　A. 1 minute.　　B. 2 minutes.　　C. 4 minutes.　　D. 8 minutes.

(7) When eating something, it is better to _____ .

　　A. eat it all at once　B. eat it slowly over time

(8) How much floss should pull out when you first start flossing?

　　A. 5 inches.　　B. 1 to 2 feet.　　C. 4 feet.

(9) Is rinsing necessary after brushing & flossing?

　　A. Yes.　　　　　B. No.

(10) When is it necessary to replace your toothbrush?

　　A. When you want a different color.

　　B. When it begins to fray.

　　C. When you win the lottery.

Writing

SCI Paper: Title Selection & Title Page

The title is perhaps the single-most important element of your research paper. It is the first thing that journal editors and reviewers see when they look at your paper and the only piece of information that fellow researchers will see in a database or search engine query.

Various categories of titles are described and each type informs readers about the content in differing manner. Generally, we will consider three broad categories: declarative, descriptive and interrogative.

Declarative titles state the main finding or conclusion stated in the paper and it is believed that a casual reader may then not have much curiosity left for reading the entire paper. Descriptive titles describe the article theme, but without divulging its findings or conclusions. Many descriptive titles include all aspects of the research question studied (participant, intervention, control and outcome; PICO). Interrogative titles usually restate the research question in part or in full. Generally, descriptive titles are preferred, as they inform the reader about what a study entails but not about the study result. This helps maintain the suspense about the outcome.

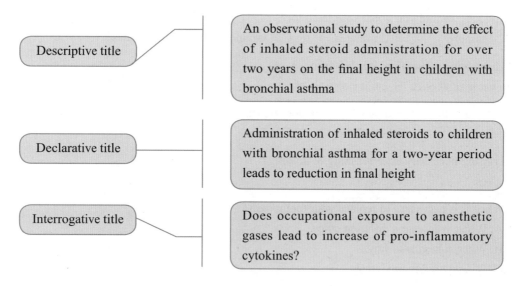

Descriptive title — An observational study to determine the effect of inhaled steroid administration for over two years on the final height in children with bronchial asthma

Declarative title — Administration of inhaled steroids to children with bronchial asthma for a two-year period leads to reduction in final height

Interrogative title — Does occupational exposure to anesthetic gases lead to increase of pro-inflammatory cytokines?

From the constructive point of view, titles can be classified as nominal, compound and full sentence titles. Nominal titles capture main premise of the study (for example, "Off-label drug use in neonatal intensive care unit"). Compound titles (or hanging titles) have a subtitle. The subtitles are primarily used to present additional relevant information. They may provide additional context, inform about the study design (for example, "Small-to-moderate decreases in cold hypersensitivity up to 3 years after severe hand injuries: A prospective cohort study") or provide geographic (for example, "Human leukocyte antigen diversity: A South African perspective") or temporal scope (for example, "Pelvic floor muscle training for female stress urinary incontinence: Five years outcomes") of the research. A subtitle is also used to add substance to a provocative or a literary (e.g., "First know thyself: cognition and error in medicine") title. Compound titles also correlate with higher number of citations. Full-sentence titles are uncommon and tend to be longer. They indicate an added degree of certainty of the study results (For example, "Serum Vitamin D Is Significantly Inversely Associated with Disease Severity in Caucasian Adults with Obstructive Sleep Apnea Syndrome"). Titles for research articles that end with an exclamatory mark are scarce.

No one construct is ideal or better than the other and they need to be chosen depending upon the article's premise. Author's individual preference and judgment also play a part.

A well-written title can function as the brand of a paper to attract editors, reviewers and readers from the very first glance, and be retrieved easily from electronic database. Generally speaking, a well-written title should be accurate, informative and concise.

☆ **Accurate**—A good title informs the reader accurately about the contents of the article. It should convey information in an unambiguous and precise manner. It should not be open to multiple interpretations and should not confuse the readers about the message it tends to communicate. To make a title accurate, it should precisely reflect the most important messages of the article and usually include key words used for indexing. It should help differentiate that particular article from other papers on the topic.

☆ **Informative**—As a condensed reflection of the paper, the title should provide enough information for the readers to know what to expect when they finish reading the whole paper.

☆ **Concise**—Short titles have more impact than long titles do, so make your title as short as possible without sacrificing accuracy and completeness. Keep in mind that the aim is to convey the topic or the message of your paper accurately, completely, specifically, and unambiguously. If you can devise a short title that fulfills these criteria, do so. Avoid using "decorative" or "empty" expressions such as "A report on," "Observations on," "Some Thought on," and "A study of."

The work on the title can begin when a paper is being written. It is a good idea to make a note of a few sentences, phrases or ideas that define the main theme of the paper; which could be later used in the title. One could go on refining these phrases, as new versions of the manuscript are written. By the time writing of the manuscript text is accomplished, the author will have a working title consisting of at least two or three key terms that can give readers a sense of the content and angle of the research paper. The next step is to compress the title by getting rid of redundant words and refining it by making it easier to read, succinct and catchy.

Title page (cover page) in submission package is the page where the title is presented, which states general information about an article including the article title, author information, any disclaimers, sources of support, etc. The following is a sample of a title page in JBR.

Available online at www.jbr-pub.org.cn

Open Access at PubMed Central

The Journal of Biomedical Research, 2019 33(3): 181–191

JBR

Original Article

Acrylamide induces HepG2 cell proliferation through upregulation of miR-21 expression

Yuyu Xu[1,Δ], Pengqi Wang[1,2,Δ], Chaoqi Xu[1], Xiaoyun Shan[1,3], Qing Feng[1,✉]

[1] *Department of Nutrition and Food Safety, School of Public Health, Nanjing Medical University, Nanjing, Jiangsu 211166, China;*
[2] *Station of Sanitary Surveillance of Lianyungang, Lianyungang, Jiangsu 222002, China;*
[3] *University of South China, Hengyang, Hunan 421000, China.*

Title:

Informative and concise;

Capitalize the first letter;

≤ 150 characters (including space);

No non-standard acronyms or abbreviations.

Author names:

Spelled out in full;

The given name first and the family name last.

Affiliations:

Provided for each author (including correspondence author) according to the order:

department/subunit, institution, city, province/state/region, postal code and country or region.

Corresponding authors annotation:

Mark with superscript using envelope symbol, including corresponding author's name, full postal address, telephone and fax numbers and e-mail address.

[Δ]These authors contributed equally to this work.

[✉]Corresponding author: Qing Feng, Department of Nutrition and Food Safety, School of Public Health, Nanjing Medical University, 101 Longmian Avenue, Nanjing, Jiangsu 211166, China. Tel: + 86-25-86868455, Email: qingfeng@njmu.edu.cn.

Received 16 February 2017, Revised 29 March 2017, Accepted 20 April 2017, Epub 27 May 2017

Acrylamide induces HepG2 proliferation by upregulating miR-21

Running title:

Describes the key meaning of the paper;

≤ 60 characters (including spaces).

Task 1

Directions: *Search the journals in your specialty to find some papers with titles of the following types.*

Nominal

_____
_____
_____
_____

Full-sentence

_____
_____
_____

Compound

_____
_____
_____

Task 2

Directions: *Rewrite the following titles to make them concise and clear and then give the reason for doing so.*

(1) Retinal arteriolar changes are an indicator of coronary artery disease

(2) Preliminary experience in using high dose of methotrexate to treat ALL

(3) A research of the relationship between the content of potassium in diet and blood pressure

(4) A retrospective study on 170 consecutive cases of abdominal pain in the emergency room

(5) A case report of SLE appearing pancreatitis and review of literatures

Task 3

Directions: *Imagine that you are researching meditation and nursing, and you draft 4 titles for you study which has shown that meditation makes nurses better communicators.*

> Title (1): Meditation Gurus
> Title (2): Why Mindful Nurses Make the Best Communicators
> Title (3): Benefits of Meditation for the Nursing Profession: A Quantitative Investigation
> Title (4): Nurses on the Move: A Quantitative Report on How Meditation Can Improve Nurse Performance

Study these titles and think about different impressions they may give.

Title _____ describes the topic and the method of the study but is not particularly catchy.

Title _____ partly describes the topic, but does not give any information about the method of the study—it could simply be a theoretical or opinion piece.

Title _____ is somewhat catchier but gives almost no information at all about the article.

Title _____ begins with a catchy main title and is followed by a subtitle that gives information about the content and method of the study.

Task 4

Directions: *The following are the footnotes on the title page of a paper. Read them and tell what they are about.*

Correspondence To: Aiqiang Xu, MD, PhD, Shandong Provincial Center for Disease Control and Prevention, 16992 Jingshi Road, Jinan, Shandong, 250014, China, Email: axuepi@163.com, or Chengbin Wang, MD, PhD, Centers for Disease Control and Prevention, 1600 Clifton Rd MS A-34, Atlanta, Georgia, 30333, USA, Email: cwang1@cdc.gov.

Word Counts: XXX in abstract, XXX in text (excluding 1 figure, 3 tables and XXX references)

Key Words: Cytomegalovirus, Seroprevalence, Congenital Infection

Financial Disclosure: The authors have no conflicts of interest to disclose.

Funding: This study was supported by a cooperative agreement between the U.S. and China CDC, and by the Taishan Scholar Program of Shandong provincial CDC.

Disclaimer: The findings and conclusions in this report are those of the authors and do not necessarily represent the official position of the Centers for Disease Control and Prevention.

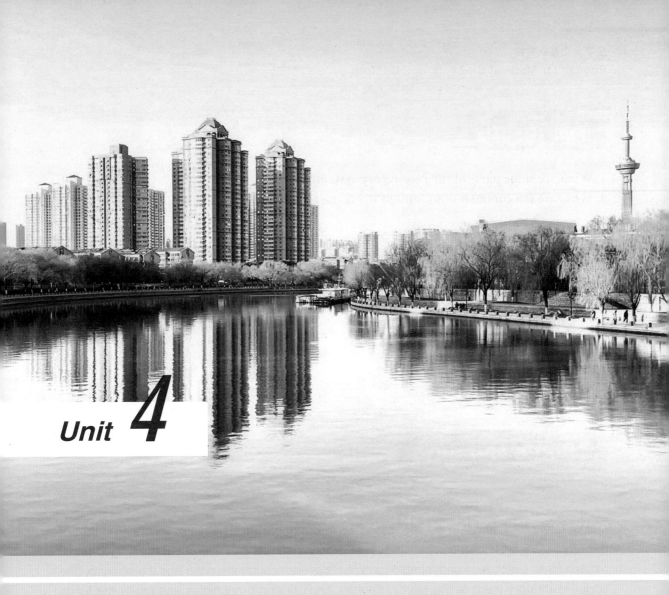

Unit *4*

The Respiratory System

√ 听力音频
√ 听力文本
√ 课件资源

Warm-up

1. **What are some parts of the respiratory system?**
2. **What are the common symptoms of the respiratory system?**

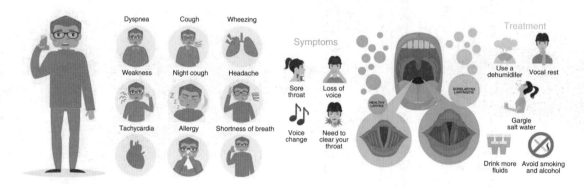

Theme Reading

The Respiratory System

We rarely think about breathing unless we're out of breath. The act of breathing is part of the respiratory system, a complex process where air travels into and out of the lungs. Air, or oxygen to be exact, plus undesirable particles, travels through the nose and the pharynx (the upper respiratory tract) to the larynx, trachea, bronchi and bronchioles and finally the lungs (the lower respiratory tract). The respiratory system is responsible for the supply of oxygen and the removal of CO_2, a process which, once interrupted for a few minutes, would surely lead to serious damage to tissues and ultimately death. Take a close look at the following text to see how the respiratory system works.

Objectives

☆ *Describe the composition of the respiratory system.*
☆ *Trace the passage through which air travels within the respiratory system.*
☆ *List the benefits of nose-breathing over mouth-breathing.*
☆ *List the defending weapons the respiratory system has against the disease-causing organisms.*
☆ *Describe the O_2-CO_2 exchange in the lungs.*

The **respiratory** system consists of organs that deliver oxygen to the circulatory system for transport to all body cells. Oxygen is essential for cells, which use this vital substance to liberate the energy needed for cellular activities. In addition to supplying oxygen, the respiratory system aids in removing of carbon dioxide, preventing the **lethal** buildup of this waste product in body tissues. Day-in and day-out, without the prompt of conscious thought, the respiratory system carries out its life-sustaining activities. If the respiratory system's tasks are interrupted for more than a few minutes, serious, and **irreversible** damage to tissues occurs, followed by the failure of all body systems, and ultimately, death.

The respiratory and circulatory systems work together to deliver oxygen to cells and remove carbon dioxide in a two-phase process called respiration. The first phase of respiration begins with breathing in, or **inhalation**. Inhalation brings air from outside the body into the lungs. Oxygen in the air moves from the lungs through blood vessels to the heart, which pumps the oxygen-rich blood to all parts of the body. Oxygen then moves from the **bloodstream** into cells, which completes the first phase of respiration. In the cells, oxygen is used in a separate energy-producing process called cellular respiration, which produces carbon dioxide as a byproduct. The second phase of respiration begins with the movement of carbon dioxide from the cells to the bloodstream. The bloodstream carries carbon dioxide to the heart, which pumps the carbon dioxide-laden blood to the lungs. In the lungs, breathing out, or **exhalation**, removes carbon dioxide from the body, thus completing the respiration cycle.

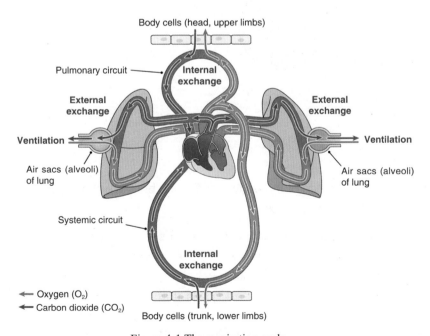

Figure 4-1 The respiration cycle

Structure

The organs of the respiratory system extend from the nose to the lungs and are divided into the upper and lower respiratory tracts. The upper respiratory tract consists of the nose and the **pharynx**, or throat. The lower respiratory tract includes the **larynx**, or voice box; the **trachea**, or windpipe, which splits into two main branches called **bronchi**; tiny branches of the bronchi called **bronchioles**; and the lungs, a pair of **saclike**, spongy organs. The nose, pharynx, larynx, trachea, bronchi and bronchioles conduct air to and from the lungs. The lungs interact with the circulatory system to deliver oxygen and remove carbon dioxide.

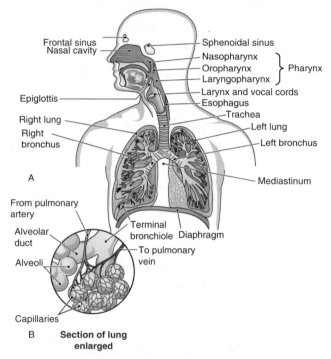

Figure 4-2 The respiratory system
A. Overview   B. Enlarged section of lung tissue

Nasal Passages

The flow of air from outside of the body to the lungs begins with the nose, which is divided into the left and right nasal passages.

The nasal passages are lined with a **membrane** composed primarily of one layer of flat, closely packed cells called epithelial cells. Each epithelial cell is densely fringed with thousands of microscopic **cilia**, fingerlike extensions of the cells. Interspersed among the **epithelial** cells are goblet cells, specialized cells that produce **mucus**, a sticky, thick, and moist fluid that coats the epithelial cells and the cilia. Numerous tiny blood vessels called **capillaries** lie just under the mucous membrane, near the surface of the nasal passages. While transporting air to the pharynx, the nasal passages play two critical roles: they filter the air to remove potentially disease-causing particles; and they moisten and warm the air to protect the structures in the respiratory system.

Filtering prevents airborne bacteria, viruses, and other potentially disease-causing substances from entering the lungs, where they may cause infection. Filtering also eliminates smog and dust particles, which may clog the narrow air passages in the smallest bronchioles. Coarse hairs found just inside the **nostrils** of the nose trap airborne particles as they are inhaled. The particles drop down onto the mucous membrane lining the nasal passages. The cilia embedded in the mucous membrane wave constantly, creating a current of mucus that propels the particles out of the nose or downward to the pharynx. In the pharynx, the mucus is swallowed and passed to the stomach, where the particles are destroyed by stomach acid. If more particles are in the nasal passages than the cilia can handle, the particles build up on the mucus and **irritate** the membrane beneath it. This irritation triggers a **reflex** that produces a sneeze to get rid of the polluted air.

The nasal passages also moisten and warm air to prevent it from damaging the delicate membranes of the lung. The mucous membranes of the nasal passages release water vapor, which moistens the air as it passes over the membranes. As air moves over the extensive capillaries in the nasal passages, it is warmed by the blood in the capillaries. If the nose is blocked or "stuffy" due to a cold or **allergies**, a person is forced to breathe through the mouth. This can be potentially harmful to the respiratory system membranes, since the mouth does not filter, warm, or moisten air.

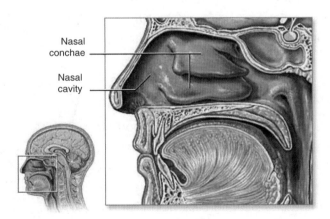

Nasal
conchae

Nasal
cavity

Figure 4-3 The nose

The Pharynx

Air leaves the nasal passages and flows to the pharynx, a short, funnel-shaped tube about 13 cm (5 inch) long that transports air to the larynx. Like the nasal passages, the pharynx is lined with a protective mucous membrane and ciliated cells that remove impurities from the air. In addition to serving as an air passage, the pharynx houses the **tonsils, lymphatic** tissues that contain white blood cells. The white blood cells attack any disease-causing organisms that escape the hairs, cilia, and mucus of the nasal passages and pharynx. In their battles with disease-causing organisms, the tonsils sometimes become swollen with infection. When the **adenoids** are swollen, they block the flow of air from the nasal passages to the pharynx and a person must breathe through the mouth.

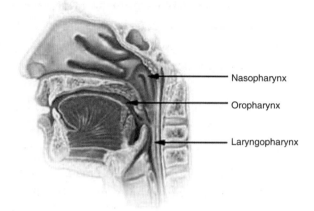

Nasopharynx

Oropharynx

Laryngopharynx

Figure 4-4 The pharynx

The Larynx

Air moves from the pharynx to the larynx, a structure about 5 cm (2 inch) long located approximately in the middle of the neck. Several layers of **cartilage**, a tough and flexible tissue, comprise most of the larynx. A protrusion in the cartilage called the Adam's apple sometimes enlarges in males during puberty, creating a prominent bulge visible on the neck.

While the primary role of the larynx is to transport air to the trachea, it also serves other functions. It plays a primary role in producing sound; it prevents food and fluid from entering the air passage to cause choking; and its mucous membranes and cilia-bearing cells help filter air. The cilia in the larynx waft airborne particles up toward the pharynx to be swallowed.

Food and fluids from the pharynx usually are prevented from entering the larynx by the **epiglottis**, a thin, leaflike

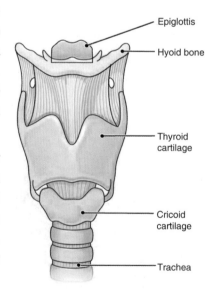

Epiglottis

Hyoid bone

Thyroid cartilage

Cricoid cartilage

Trachea

Figure 4-5 The larynx

tissue. The "stem" of the leaf attaches to the front and top of the larynx. When a person is breathing, the epiglottis is held in a vertical position, like an open trap door. When a person swallows, however, a reflex causes the larynx and the epiglottis to move toward each other, forming a protective seal, and food and fluids are routed to the esophagus. If a person is eating or drinking too rapidly, or laughs while swallowing, the swallowing reflex may not work, and food or fluid can enter the larynx. Food, fluid, or other substances in the larynx initiate a cough reflex as the body attempts to clear the larynx of the obstruction.

The Trachea, Bronchi and Bronchioles

Air passes from the larynx into the trachea, a tube about 12 to 15 cm (about 5 to 6 inch) long located just below the larynx. The trachea is formed of 15 to 20 C-shaped rings of cartilage. The sturdy cartilage rings hold the trachea open, enabling air to pass freely at all times. The open part of the C-shaped cartilage lies at the back of the trachea and the ends of the "C" are connected by muscle tissue.

The base of the trachea is located a little below where the neck meets the trunk of the body. Here the trachea branches into two tubes, the left and right bronchi, which deliver air to the left and right lungs, respectively. Within the lungs, the bronchi branch into smaller tubes called bronchioles. The trachea, bronchi and the first few bronchioles contribute to the cleansing function of the respiratory system, for they, too, are lined with mucous membranes and ciliated cells that move mucus upward to the pharynx.

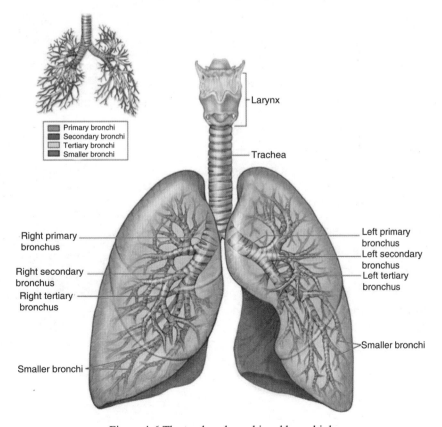

Figure 4-6 The trachea, bronchi and bronchioles

The Alveoli

The bronchioles divide many more times in the lungs to create an impressive tree with smaller and smaller branches, some no larger than 0.5 mm (0.02 in) in diameter. These branches dead-end into tiny air sacs called **alveoli**. The alveoli deliver oxygen to the circulatory system and remove carbon dioxide. Interspersed among the alveoli are numerous **macrophages**, large white blood cells that patrol the alveoli and remove foreign substances that have not been filtered out earlier. The macrophages are the last line of defense of the respiratory system; their presence helps ensure that the alveoli are protected from infection so that they can carry out their vital role.

The alveoli number about 150 million per lung and comprise most of the lung tissue. Alveoli resemble tiny, collapsed balloons with thin elastic walls that expand as air flows into them and collapse when the air is exhaled. Alveoli are arranged in grapelike clusters, and each cluster is surrounded by a dense hairnet of tiny, thin-walled capillaries. The alveoli and capillaries are arranged in such a way that air in the wall of the alveoli is only about 0.1 to 0.2 microns from the blood in the capillary. Since the concentration of oxygen is much higher in the alveoli than in the capillaries, the oxygen diffuses from the alveoli to the capillaries. The oxygen flows through the capillaries to larger vessels, which carry the oxygenated blood to the heart, where it is pumped to the rest of the body.

Carbon dioxide that has been dumped into the bloodstream as a waste product from cells throughout the body flows through the bloodstream to the heart, and then to the alveolar capillaries. The concentration of carbon dioxide in the capillaries is much higher than in the alveoli, causing carbon dioxide to **diffuse** into the alveoli. Exhalation forces the carbon dioxide back through the respiratory passages and then to the outside of the body.

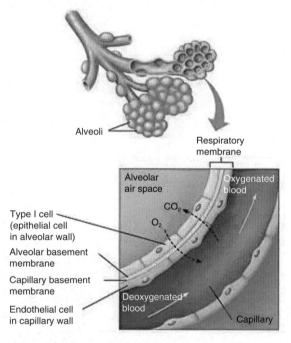

Figure 4-7 The alveoli

Vocabulary

adenoid [ˈædɪnɔɪd]　a collection of lymphatic tissue in the throat behind the uvula (on the posterior wall and roof of the nasopharynx)

alveolus [ælˈviːələs]　a tiny sac for holding air in the lungs, formed by the terminal dilation of tiny air passageways

allergy [ˈælədʒi]　hypersensitivity reaction to a particular allergen

bloodstream [ˈblʌdˌstriːm]　the blood flowing through the circulatory system

bronchiole [ˈbrɒŋkɪəʊl]　any of the smallest bronchial ducts, ending in alveoli

bronchus [ˈbrɒŋkəs]　(pl. bronchi) either of the two main branches of the trachea

capillary [kəˈpɪləri]　any of the minute blood vessels connecting arterioles with venules

cartilage [ˈkɑːtɪlɪdʒ]　tough elastic tissue, mostly converted to bone in adults

cilia [ˈsɪlɪə]　the fine hairlike projections from certain cells such as those in the respiratory tract that sweep in unison and help to sweep away fluids and particles

diffuse [dɪˈfjuːs]　to spread out over a large space

epiglottis [ˌepɪˈglɒtɪs]　a flap of cartilage that covers the windpipe while swallowing

epithelial [ˌepɪˈθiːlɪəl]　of or belonging to the epithelium

exhalation [ˌekshəˈleɪʃən]　the act of expelling air from the lungs

inhalation [ˌɪnhəˈleɪʃən]　the drawing in of air (or other gases) as in breathing

irreversible [ɪrɪˈvɜːsəbl]　impossible to change back to a previous condition or state

irritate [ˈɪrɪteɪt]　to make (part of your body) sore or painful

larynx [ˈlærɪŋks]　a cartilaginous structure at the top of the trachea, containing elastic vocal cords that are the source of the vocal tone in speech

lethal [ˈliːθəl]　capable of causing death

lymphatic [ˌlɪmˈfætɪk]　of or relating to or produced by lymph

macrophage [ˈmækrəʊfeɪdʒ]　a large phagocyte either fixing or circulating in the blood stream

membrane [ˈmembreɪn]　a pliable sheet of tissue that covers or lines or connects organs or cells of animals

mucus [ˈmjuːkəs]　protective secretion of the mucous membranes, which lubricates the passage of food and protects the epithelial cells in the gut, making it difficult for bacteria to penetrate the body through the epitheliumin of the nose and throat and lungs

nostril [ˈnɒstrɪl]　either one of the two external openings to the nasal cavity in the nose

pharynx [ˈfærɪŋks]　the passage to the stomach and lungs, in the front part of the neck below the chin and above the collarbone

reflex [ˈriːfleks]　an automatic instinctive unlearned reaction to a stimulus

respiratory [ˈrespərətəri; riˈspaɪə-]　pertaining to respiration

saclike [ˈsæklaɪk]　shaped like a pouch

tonsil [ˈtʌnsɪl]　either of two masses of lymphatic tissue one on each side of the oral pharynx

trachea [ˈtreɪkɪə]　membranous tube with cartilaginous rings that conveys inhaled air from the larynx to the bronchi

Task 1

Directions: *Select the letter of the choice that best completes the statement or answers the question.*

(1) The organs of the respiratory system deliver oxygen to the _____ system for transport to all body cells.

    A. muscular   B. digestive   C. circulatory   D. reproductive

(2) External exchange takes place in the _____, located in the thoracic cavity.

    A. nose   B. pharynx   C. mouth   D. lungs

(3) Air passes through the nasal cavity, where foreign bodies are _____.

    A. moistened   B. warmed up   C. filtered out   D. irritated

(4) The respiratory tract is moist with _____ and lined with ____ that sweep particles out of the airways.

    A. surfactant; cells   B. fluid; squamous tissue

    C. surfactant; cartilage   D. mucus; cilia

(5) The membrane around the lungs is the _____ .

    A. peritoneum   B. pleura   C. mucosa   D. mediatinum

(6) As expelled air passes the _____, they vibrate to produce sounds.

    A. pharynx   B. vocal cords   C. Adam's apple   D. glottis

(7) What prevents food or drink from entering the trachea during swallowing?

    A. Esophagus.   B. Palatine.   C. Tonsil.   D. Epiglottis.

(8) What are the tubes that carry air from the trachea into the lungs?

    A. vessels   B. nares   C. diaphragm   D. bronchi

(9) It is through the ultra thin walls of the _____ and their surrounding capillaries that oxygen diffuses into the blood and carbon dioxide diffuses out of the blood for elimination.

    A. diaphragm   B. alveoli   C. villi   D. pleura

(10) The amount of _____ that is exhaled is important in regulating the blood's acidity or alkalinity, based on the amount of carbonic acid that is formed.

    A. oxygen   B. hemoglobin   C. carbon dioxide   D. red blood cell

Task 2

Directions: *Label the organs of the respiratory system.*

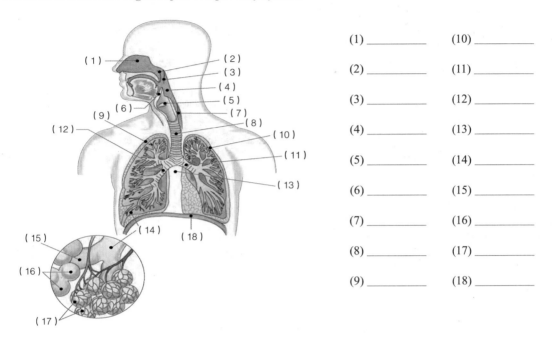

(1) _____	(10) _____
(2) _____	(11) _____
(3) _____	(12) _____
(4) _____	(13) _____
(5) _____	(14) _____
(6) _____	(15) _____
(7) _____	(16) _____
(8) _____	(17) _____
(9) _____	(18) _____

Task 3

Directions: *Fill in the following table based on the text above or relevant information from the Internet and then talk about the respiratory process.*

Structure	Function
(1) nasal passages	
(2) goblet cells	
(3) cilia	
(4) pharynx	
(5) tonsils	
(6) larynx	
(7) trachea	
(8) bronchi	
(9) bronchioles	
(10) alveoli	

Task 4

Directions: *Match each of the following terms in Column A with its definition in Column B.*

A	B
(1) pharynx	A. the enlarged, superior portion of the trachea that contains the vocal cords

(to be continued)

(2) inspiration	B. the air passageway that extends from the larynx to the bronchi
(3) trachea	C. the space between the lungs together with the organs contained in this space
(4) larynx	D. the act of drawing air into the lungs; inhalation
(5) vocal cords	E. the throat; a common passageway for food entering the esophagus and air entering the larynx
(6) alveoli	F. a cone-shaped, spongy respiratory organ contained within the thorax
(7) lung	G. branches of the windpipe that lead into the lungs
(8) mediastinum	H. membranous folds on either side of the larynx that are important in speech production, also called vocal folds
(9) cilia	I. thin hairs attached to the mucous membrane lining the respiratory tract
(10) bronchi	J. air sacs of the lung

Medical Terminology

Roots	Terminology	Term Analysis	Definition
nose			
nas(o) [ˈneɪzəʊ]	nasal [ˈneɪzəl] nasitis [neɪˈsaɪtɪs]		
rhin(o) [ˈraɪnəʊ]	rhinorrhea [raɪnəʊˈriːə] rhinoplasty [ˌraɪnəʊˈplæsti]	-rrhea=discharge, flow	
pharynx / throat			
pharyng(o) [ˈfærɪŋəʊ] pharynge- [ˈfærɪndʒi]	pharyngitis [ˌfærɪnˈdʒaɪtɪs] pharyngoscopy [ˌfærɪŋˈɡɒskəpi]		
tonsils			
tonsill(o) [ˈtɒnsɪləʊ]	peritonsillar [ˌperɪˈtɒnsɪlə] tonsillectomy [ˌtɒnsɪˈlektəmi]	peri-=around	
epiglottis			
epiglott(o) [epɪˈɡlɒtəʊ]	epiglottitis [epɪɡlɒˈtaɪtɪs] epiglottal [ˌepɪˈɡlɒtəl]		
trachea / windpipe			

(to be continued)

trache(o) ['treɪkɪəʊ]	tracheostomy [ˌtreɪkɪ'ɒstəmi] tracheitis [ˌtreɪkɪ'aɪtɪs]	-stomy=forming an opening (mouth)	
larynx / voice box			
laryng(o) [lə'rɪŋgəʊ]	laryngoscope [lə'rɪŋgəskəʊp] laryngitis [ˌlærɪn'dʒaɪtɪs]	-scope=instrument for examining	
bronchus (pl. bronchi)			
bronch(o) ['brɒŋkəʊ] bronchi(o) ['brɒŋkɪəʊ]	bronchoscopy [brɒŋ'kɒskəpi] bronchiectasis [brɒŋkɪ'ektəsɪs]	-ectasis=dilation, expansion	
bronchiole			
bronchiol(o) ['brɒŋkɪəʊləʊ]	bronchiolitis [ˌbrɒŋkɪəʊ'laɪtɪs] bronchiole ['brɒŋkɪəʊl]		
air; lung			
pneum(o) ['nju:məʊ] pneumon(o) ['nju:məʊnəʊ]	pneumectomy [nju:'mektəmi] pneumonia [nju:'məʊnɪə]		
lung			
pulm(o) ['pʌlməʊ] pulmon(o) ['pʌlməʊnəʊ]	pulmonologist [pʌlmə'nɒlədʒɪst] pulmonitis [pʌlməʊ'naɪtɪs]	-logist=specialist in study of	
chest			
thorac(o) ['θɔ:rəkəʊ]	thoracopathy [ˌθɔ:rə'kɒpəθi] thoracocentesis [ˌθɔ:rəkəʊsen'ti:sɪs]	-pathy=disease	
pector(o) ['pektərəʊ]	pectoral ['pektərəl] expectoration [ɪkˌspektə'reɪʃn]		
breathing			
pne(o) ['pnɪəʊ]	apnea [æp'nɪə] bradypnea [bræ'dɪpnɪə]	a-=without, not	

(to be continued)

spir(o) [ˈspaɪərəʊ]	spirometer [ˌspaɪəˈrɒmɪtə] spiroscope [ˈspaɪərəskəʊp]		
alveolus, air sac			
alveol(o) [ælˈvɪələʊ]	alveolar [ælˈvɪələ] alveolitis [ˌælvɪəˈlaɪtɪs]		
pleura			
pleur(o) [ˈplʊərəʊ]	pleurodynia [ˌplʊərəˈdɪnɪə] pleurocholecystitis [plʊərəʊˌkəʊlɪsɪsˈtaɪtɪs]	odyn(o)=pain	
straight, upright			
orth(o) [ˈɔːθəʊ]	orthodontia [ˌɔːθəʊˈdɒnʃɪə] orthopnea [ˌɔːθɒpˈniːə]	odont(o)=tooth	
oxygen			
ox(o) [ˈɒksəʊ] oxi- [ˈɒksi] oxy- [ˈɒksi]	hypoxia [haɪˈpɒksɪə] oxide [ˈɒksaɪd]	hypo-=under, below, deficient	
blue			
cyan(o) [ˈsaɪənəʊ]	cyanosis [ˌsaɪəˈnəʊsɪs] cyanopsia [ˌsaɪəˈnɒpsɪə]		
lobe of the lung			
lob(o) [ˈləʊbəʊ]	lobectomy [ləʊˈbektəmi] lobulus [ˈlɒbjuːləs]	-tomy=surgical removal	
mediastinum			
mediastin(o) [miːdɪəsˈtaɪnəʊ]	mediastinoscopy [ˌmiːdɪˌæstɪˈnɒskəpi] mediastinum [ˌmiːdɪəsˈtaɪnəm]		
diaphragm			
phren(o) [ˈfrenəʊ]	phrenic [ˈfrenɪk] phrenitis [frɪˈnaɪtɪs]		

(to be continued)

voice			
phon(o) [ˈfəʊnəʊ]	dysphonia [dɪsˈfəʊnɪə] aphonia [əˈfəʊnɪə]	dys-=difficult	
carbon dioxide			
capn(o) [ˈkæpnəʊ]	hypercapnia [ˌhaɪpəˈkæpnɪə] capnophilic [kæpnəʊˈfɪlɪk]	phil(o)=love, affinity	
gland			
aden(o) [ˈædɪnəʊ]	adenoids [ˈædɪnɔɪdz] adenoidectomy [ˌædɪnɔɪˈdektəmɪ]	-oid=resembling	
sinus			
sin(o) [ˈsaɪnəʊ] sinu [ˈsaɪnju]	sinobronchitis [saɪnəʊbrɒnˈkaɪtɪs] perisinusitis [ˌperɪˌsaɪnjuˈsaɪtɪs]	peri-=around, surrounding	
spitting			
pty(o) [taɪəʊ] ptys- [tɪs]	hemoptysis [hɪˈmɒptɪsɪs] plasmoptysis [plæzˈmɒptɪsɪs]	hem(o)=blood	
narrowing			
sten(o) [ˈstɪnəʊ]	dacryostenosis [dækrɪəʊstɪˈnəʊsɪs] rectostenosis [ˌrektəʊstɪˈnəʊsɪs]	dacry(o)=tears	
dilatation			
ectas [ˈektəs]	arteriectasis [ˌɑːtərɪˈektəsɪs] venectasia [ˌviːnekˈteɪzɪə]	arteri(o)=artery	
air			
aer(o) [ˈeərəʊ] aeri- [ˈeəri]	aerobic [eəˈrəʊbɪk] aerophagia [eərəˈfeɪdʒɪə]	phag(o)=swallowing	

(to be continued)

pus			
py(o) ['paɪəʊ] py ['paɪ]	pyogenesis [ˌpaɪəʊˈdʒenɪsɪs] pyometra [ˌpaɪəʊˈmiːtrə]	gen(o)=producing, coming to be metr(o)=uterus	
smelling			
osm(o) ['ɒzməʊ]	anosmia [æˈnɒzmjə] osmology [ɒzˈmɒlədʒi]		
cartilage; granules			
chondr(o) ['kɒndrəʊ]	chondromalacia [ˌkɒndrəʊməˈleɪʃə] chondrify ['kɒndrɪfaɪ] mitochondrion [ˌmaɪtəʊˈkɒndriən]	malac(o)=softening	
mucus			
muc(o) ['mjuːkəʊ] muci ['mjuːsɪ]	mucin ['mjuːsɪn] mucigenous [mjuːˈsɪdʒɪnəs]	-in=agent	

Vocabulary Study

Task 1

Directions: *Match each of the following terms with its definition and underline the strong part of each word where there are two or more syllables.*

(1) hypercapnemia	A. chronic dilation of a bronchus
(2) hypopnea	B. increased carbon dioxide in the blood
(3) cyanosis	C. decreased rate and depth of breathing
(4) bronchiectasis	D. condition of blueness of skin
(5) pleuritis	E. inflammation of pleura

(6) rhinoplasty	A. removal of a region of a lung
(7) thoracoscopy	B. surgical puncture of the chest
(8) pneumonectomy	C. surgical repair of the nose
(9) thoracentesis	D. incision of the trachea through the neck
(10) tracheotomy	E. endoscopic examination of the chest

Task 2

Directions: *Fill in the blanks with appropriate words for body parts.*

(1) The double membrane that covers the lungs and lines the thoracic cavity is the _____.

(2) The small air sacs in the lungs through which gases are exchanged between the atmosphere and the blood are the _____.

(3) The trachea divides into a right and a left primary _____.

(4) A pneumotropic virus is one that invades the _____.

(5) Thoracentesis is a word for surgical puncture of the _____.

(6) A tracheostomy is the creation of an opening into the _____.

(7) A bronchostenosis is the narrowing of a _____.

(8) A person who has bronchiolitis has an inflammation of the _____.

(9) Epiglottitis means inflammation of the _____ that may lead to upper airway obstruction .

(10) Rhinoplasty is a word for the plastic repair of the _____.

(11) During a tonsillectomy, a removal of lymph tissue is made in the _____.

(12) Laryngectomy is a word for the removal of the _____.

(13) Mediastinoscopy means an examination of the _____ by means of an endoscope inserted through an incision above the sternum.

(14) Nasal cannula is a two-pronged plastic device inserted into the _____ for delivery of oxygen.

(15) Adenoidectomy is a word for a surgical removal of the _____.

Task 3

Directions: *Write a word for each of the following definitions using the word parts provided.*

| intra- | -tomy | nas(o) | pleur(o) | -ia | -al |
| pharynge- | pne(o) | trache(o) | eu- | -a | alg(o)- |

(1) pain in the pleura _____

(2) easy, normal breathing _____

(3) within the nose _____

(4) pertaining to the pharynx _____

(5) surgical incision of the trachea _____

-osis	-plasty	phon(o)	-ectomy	cyan(o)	-ia
a-	tonsill(o)	rhin(o)	-centesis	thorac(o)	

(6) condition of blueness of skin _____

(7) removal of lymph tissue in the oropharynx _____

(8) surgical repair of the nose _____

(9) surgical puncture of the chest to remove fluid from the pleural space _____

(10) loss of the voice _____

pneumon(o)	bronchiol(o)	capn(o)	hyper-	ox(o)	-is
ectas(o)	laryng(o)	spasm(o)	hypo-	-ia	

(11) sudden contraction of the larynx _____

(12) dilatation of the bronchioles _____

(13) inflammation of the lung _____

(14) decreased amount of oxygen in the tissues _____

(15) increased carbon dioxide in the tissues_____

Case Study 4-1

Terminal Dyspnea

N.A., a 76-YO woman, was in the ICU in the terminal stage of multisystem organ failure. She had been admitted to the hospital for bacterial pneumonia, which had not resolved with antibiotic therapy. She had a 20-year history of COPD. She was not conscious and was unable to breathe on her own. Her ABGs were abnormal, and she was diagnosed with refractory ARDS. The decision was made to support her breathing with endotracheal intubation and mechanical ventilation. After one week and several unsuccessful attempts to wean her from the ventilator, the pulmonologist suggested a permanent tracheostomy and discussed with the family the options of continuing or withdrawing life support. Her physiologic status met the criteria of remote or no chance for recovery.

N.A.'s family discussed her condition and decided not to pursue aggressive life-sustaining therapies. N.A. was assigned DNR status. After the written orders were read and signed by the family, the endotracheal tube, feeding tube, pulse oximeter, and ECG electrodes were removed, and a morphine IV drip was started with prn boluses ordered to promote comfort and relieve pain. The family sat with her for many hours, providing comfort and support. After a while, they noticed that her breathing had become shallow with Cheyne-Stokes respirations. N.A. died quietly in the presence of her family and the hospital chaplain.

Task 4

Directions: *Select the best answer to the question or the statement based on the information provided in the case of terminal dyspnea.*

(1) What's the patient's physical condition when she was in the ICU?

    A. The patient's vital signs was stable.

    B. The patient's condition was undetermined.

    C. The patient was critical, and even death is possible.

    D. The patient was conscious. However, there may be minor complications.

(2) The patient had been admitted to the hospital with _____.

    A. tuberculous pleuritis   B. allergic asthma

    C. chronic bronchitis   D. bacterial pneumonia

(3) COPD, abbreviation for _____, is a progressive disease that makes it hard to breathe.

    A. coronary obstruction pulmonary disease

    B. chronic obstructive pulmonary disease

    C. comprehensive operation planning directive

    D. cystic oral pneumonia disease

(4) ABG(s) is a blood test that is performed using blood from a(an) _____.

    A. aorta   B. vein   C. capillary   D. artery

(5) The term "refractory" refers to _____.

    A. temporarily responsive to drugs

    B. not responding to treatment

    C. fully responsive to nervous stimuli

    D. responding to authority

(6) Endotracheal intubation may be used as an emergency measure when _____ are blocked.

    A. body cavities B. adenoids   C. vessels   D. airways

(7) An endotracheal tube is placed _____.

    A. within the trachea   B. within the bronchus

    C. around the airway   D. under the trachea

(8) Tracheostomy can be used to prepare for the insertion of a tube for _____.

    A. digestion   B. metabolism   C. ventilation   D. blood circulation

(9) Pulse oximetry is used to measure _____.

    A. forced expiratory volume

    B. tidal volume

C. positive end-expiratory pressure

D. oxygen saturation of blood

(10) Dyspnea could NOT be described as _____.

    A. difficulty in breathing   B. normal respiration

    C. labored breathing   D. shortness of breath

Case Study 4-2

Thoracentesis

A 22-year-old known heroin abuser was admitted to an emergency department comatose with shallow respirations. Routine laboratory studies and chest X-ray studies were done after the patient was aroused. He was then transferred to the ICU. He complained of left-sided chest pain. Examination of the chest X-ray showed three fractured ribs on the right and a large right pleural effusion. Further questioning of a friend revealed that he had fallen and struck the corner of a table after injecting heroin. The diagnosis was traumatic hemothorax secondary to rib fractures.

Description of Procedure In pleural effusion, other materials accumulate in the pleural space. Depending on the substance involved, these are described as empyema (pyothorax); hemothorax; or hydrothorax. Causes of these conditions include injury, infection, heart failure, and pulmonary embolism. Thoracentesis may be required to obtain pleural fluid for diagnosis or to therapeutically drain a pleural effusion, which is performed as follows:

Bedside Ultrasonography After the patient has been positioned, ultrasonography is performed to confirm the pleural effusion, assess its size, look for loculations, determine the optimal puncture site, improve the administration of local anesthetics, and, most important, minimize the complications of the procedure.

Preparation of Puncture Site The patient is sitting in the correct position for the procedure; it allows the chest wall to be pulled outward in an expanded position. A wide area is cleaned with an antiseptic bacteriostatic solution. The skin, subcutaneous tissue, rib periosteum, intercostal muscles, and parietal pleura should be well infiltrated with anesthetic.

Insertion of Device or Catheter and Drainage of Effusion With aspiration initiated, the device is advanced over the superior aspect of the rib until pleural fluid is obtained. The needle is inserted close to the base of the effusion so that gravity can help with drainage, but it is kept as far away from the diaphragm as possible.

Completion of Procedure The catheter or needle is carefully removed, and the wound is dressed. The patient is repositioned as appropriate for his or her comfort and respiratory status.

Task 5

Directions: *Write a word or phrase from the case study that means the same as each of the following.*

(1) the surgical puncture of the pleural cavity using a hollow needle, in order to withdraw fluid, drain blood, etc _____

(2) the presence of pus in a body cavity, especially the pleural cavity _____

(3) the technique of using ultrasound to produce pictures of structures within the body _____

(4) a drug that causes temporary loss of bodily sensations _____

(5) an exudate of fluid into the pleural cavity _____

(6) a medical problem that occurs as a result of another illness or disease _____

(7) a thick fibrous two-layered membrane covering the surface of bones _____

(8) accumulation of blood in the pleural cavity _____

(9) an accumulation of fluid in one or both pleural cavities, often resulting from disease of the heart or kidneys _____

(10) removal of air or fluid from a body cavity by suction _____

Medical Term Extension

Guidelines on Personal Protective Equipment (PPE)

The selection of PPE depends on medical hazards. Contact with blood and/or saliva requires PPE. In dental clinics, primary PPE is as follows:

☆ Disposable surgical gloves
☆ Disposable surgical masks
☆ Goggles
☆ Face shields

These items protect medical staff from contaminants. Dentists and hygienists are at risk for infectious diseases. To prevent further contamination, properly dispose of PPE.

The following provides the procedure for the removal of PPE:

☆ First, remove surgical gloves.
☆ Next, remove face shields/goggles.
☆ Finally, remove surgical masks.

Place goggles and face shields in dispensers. They are reusable.

Be sure to wash your hands immediately afterwards. Use antibacterial soap and warm water. Lather hands and rub for one minute. Then, rinse.

Task 6

Directions: *Name the following items in English.*

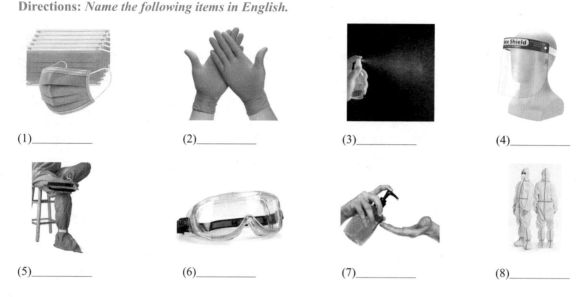

(1)_____   (2)_____   (3)_____   (4)_____

(5)_____   (6)_____   (7)_____   (8)_____

Task 7

Directions: *Read the following advertisement. Then discuss what equipment an EMS worker uses to treat a fracture.*

Attention,
EMS managers!
Do you need affordable, high-quality equipment? Call TCO Medical Supply!
We carry a full range of supplies for wound dressings. You'll find bandages and tape in a variety of sizes. Plus, our gloves and masks reliably protect paramedics from exposure to infectious agents. Also, check out our line of precision tools. We carry scissors, needles, and many other instruments.

Do you handle musculoskeletal injuries? Immobilize the area with the right splint or cervical collar. All ambulances and ERs need reliable equipment for moving injured patients. That's why we also have a wide selection of wheelchairs and gurneys. And don't forget stiff boards for those tricky spinal injuries.

Writing

Medical Abstract (I)

The abstract is a concise statement of the major elements of your paper. It is usually the last section written by the authors, but is the first section of your paper that is read by the editors and reviewers. It should therefore provide a snapshot of the research undertaken by you. In addition, it should be comprehensive yet crisp. The abstract should highlight the selling point of your research work and should lure the readers to read the whole paper. Besides determining selection of the paper, abstracts are also important for indexing. When searching online for research work, most databases would display the title as well as the abstract. This would enable the readers to determine if they really need to go through the full text of your research paper. However, it is important to remember that for your article to be picked up during an online search, it must contain the key words that a potential researcher would use to search.

What Should the Abstract Contain?

The abstract should be a window to your research and should effectively convey all the elements of the research work. The abstract essentially has four elements (BOX 1).

BOX 1 Elements of the abstract

Purpose	Why this work? What was aimed?
Methods	How was it achieved?
Results	What are the findings?
Conclusion	What is the inference?

Abstracts cover all the aspects of the research including the background, objectives, methods, results, conclusions, and recommendations. They, however, do not provide a critique of the research. These are usually around 300 words or about 10% of the length of the manuscript.

Format of an Abstract

Abstract can be written in running text without the use of subheadings (Unstructured abstract) or it may be in a structured format with use of subheadings. A structured abstract may be a 4-point abstract

BOX 2 Subheadings of a 4-point abstract

(1) Background and/or Objectives
(2) Methods
(3) Results
(4) Conclusions

or a detailed traditional 8-point abstract. You will have to choose the format of the abstract after checking the "Instructions to Authors" of the journal you wish to submit your research to.

The 4-point abstract is easy to write as the elements are distinct entities. They are:

Background—It should be brief and limited to two or three sentences, where you need to specify what is already known and why you conducted the study. The objectives of study should also be mentioned.

Methods—This is usually the longest section of the abstract and should give enough information to the readers to understand what was your work and how was your study done. The important aspects that need to be covered here include the study design, study setting, clinical diagnosis of participants, sample size calculation, sampling methods, intervention done, duration of the study, research instruments used, and the primary and secondary outcome measures and how these were assessed.

Results—This is the most important and difficult section to write in an abstract. The results should mention the exact number of participants including the dropouts, and adverse effects, if any. The results of the analysis of the primary objectives and the salient secondary objectives should be presented in words as well as numbers including P values. An abstract should present the results of your research as data (mean, standard deviation, 95% confidence interval, mean difference, P value, median, and interquartile range, where applicable). Merely stating the interpretation of results in sentences without numerical results is inappropriate.

Conclusions—The conclusions need to state the "take home message" and any other salient findings which need to be considered. The conclusions must always take into account your hypothesis and research question and must be written so as to answer the same in the light of your results. Additionally, you may present your perspective in this section of the abstract.

Here is an example:

Persistence of Zika Virus in Body Fluids
— Final Report

BACKGROUND
To estimate the frequency and duration of detectable Zika virus (ZIKV) RNA in human body fluids, we prospectively assessed a cohort of recently infected participants in Puerto Rico.

METHODS
We evaluated samples obtained from 295 participants (including 94 men who provided semen specimens) in whom ZIKV RNA was detected on reverse-transcriptase–polymerase-chain-reaction (RT-PCR) assay in urine or blood at an enhanced arboviral clinical surveillance site. We collected serum, urine, saliva, semen, and vaginal secretions weekly for the first month and at 2, 4, and 6 months. All specimens were tested by means of RT-PCR, and serum was

tested with the use of anti–ZIKV IgM enzyme-linked immunosorbent assay. Among the participants with ZIKV RNA in any specimen at week 4, collection continued every 2 weeks thereafter until all specimens tested negative. We used parametric Weibull regression models to estimate the time until the loss of ZIKV RNA detection in each body fluid and reported the findings in medians and 95th percentiles.

RESULTS

The medians and 95th percentiles for the time until the loss of ZIKV RNA detection were 15 days (95% confidence interval [CI], 14 to 17) and 41 days (95% CI, 37 to 44), respectively, in serum; 11 days (95% CI, 9 to 12) and 34 days (95% CI, 30 to 38) in urine; and 42 days (95% CI, 35 to 50) and 120 days (95% CI, 100 to 139) in semen. Less than 5% of participants had detectable ZIKV RNA in saliva or vaginal secretions.

CONCLUSIONS

The prolonged time until ZIKV RNA clearance in serum in this study may have implications for the diagnosis and prevention of ZIKV infection. In 95% of the men in this study, ZIKV RNA was cleared from semen after approximately 4 months.

The 8-point abstract ensures completion of all aspects of the research; however, there is a significant overlap between the Methods and Results section. Therefore, it needs to be drafted very carefully. For example, under the subheading "participants", you will not only need to specify the inclusion/exclusion criteria (part of methods section), but also need to mention the exact number recruited in your study (part of results).

BOX 3 Subheadings of an 8-point abstract

(1) Objectives
(2) Design
(3) Setting
(4) Participants
(5) Methods/ Intervention
(6) Outcome measures
(7) Results
(8) Conclusions

Here is an example:

Vitamin D Supplementation for Severe Pneumonia — A Randomized Controlled Trial

Objective: To determine the role of oral vitamin D supplementation for resolution of severe pneumonia in under-five children.

Design: Randomized, double blind, placebo-controlled trial.

Setting: Inpatients from a tertiary care hospital.

Participants: Two hundred children [mean (SD) age: 13.9 (11.7) months; boys: 120] between 2 months to 5 years with severe pneumonia. Pneumonia was diagnosed in the presence of fever, cough, tachypnea (as per WHO cut-offs) and crepitations. Children with pneumonia and chest indrawing or at least one of the danger sign (inability to feed, lethargy, cyanosis) were diagnosed as having severe pneumonia. The two groups were comparable for baseline characteristics including age, anthropometry, socio-demographic profile, and clinical and laboratory parameters.

Intervention: Oral vitamin D (1000 IU for <1 year and 2000 IU for >1 year) (n=100) or placebo (lactose) (n=100) once a day for 5 days, from enrolment. Both the groups received antibiotics as per the Indian Academy of Pediatrics guidelines, and supportive care (oxygen, intravenous fluids and monitoring).

Outcome variables: Primary: time to resolution of severe pneumonia. Secondary: duration of hospitalization and time to resolution of tachypnea, chest retractions and inability to feed.

Results: Median duration (SE, 95% CI) of resolution of severe pneumonia was similar in the two groups [vitamin D: 72 (3.7, 64.7-79.3) hours; placebo: 64 (4.5, 55.2-72.8) hours]. Duration of hospitalization and time to resolution of tachypnea, chest retractions, and inability to feed were also comparable between the two groups.

Conclusion: Short-term supplementation with oral vitamin D (1000-2000 IU per day for 5 days) has no beneficial effect on resolution of severe pneumonia in under-five children. Further studies need to be conducted with higher dose of Vitamin D or longer duration of supplementation to corroborate these findings.

Task 1

Directions: *Choose a proper subheading for each sentence of the abstract below.*

(A) To construct a reference range of SpO2 values in healthy preterm infants using a simple data logging device. (B) Thirty-three healthy preterm infants were monitored for a continuous period of 4 hours at rest using an Ohmeda Biox 3700 E Pulse Oximeter and an electronic data logger (Rustrack Ranger). (C) Stored data were downloaded and saved as individual files on a personal computer. (D) The study group median and 5th and 95th percentiles were used to construct a cumulative frequency curve of time against SpO2 value, representing the normal reference range of SpO2 profiles in healthy preterm infants. (E) Comparison of an infant's SpO2 profile against this curve may be more helpful in guiding supplemental oxygen treatment in that individual than a figure for a mean SpO2 and its standard deviation.

Task 2

Directions: *The following disordered sentences are taken from a 4-point abstract. Rearrange these sentences in their correct order.*

A. Incidence of lung cancer in exposed workers ranked the first place, with an SMR of 2.648, as compared with that of non-exposed workers. Incidence of lung cancer in the dust-exposed workers with a longer duration of employment was significantly higher than in those with a shorter one. Incidence of lung cancer in exposed workers with a wet operation mode was lower than that in those with dry-operation mode.

B. A retrospective cohort study was conducted in 16711 workers exposed to dust and 7598 non-exposed workers.

C. Malignant tumor, especially lung cancer, occurred more frequently in the workers exposed to dust, which could be a potential risk factor contributing to carcinogenesis.

D. To investigate incidence of malignant tumor in workers exposed to dust in a mine during the past 30 years.

Background/Objective _____

Method _____

Result _____

Conclusion _____

Task 3

Directions: *The following disordered sentences are taken from an abstract, entitled Childhood Vaccines and Antibiotic Use in Low-and middle-income Countries (Lewnard JA, Nature, 2020). Rearrange these sentences into a well-organized non-structured abstract by numbering them from 1 to 10.*

A. Here we show that vaccines that have recently been implemented in the World Health Organization's Expanded Programme on Immunization reduce antibiotic consumption substantially among children under five years of age in LMICs.

B. Under current coverage levels, pneumococcal and rotavirus vaccines prevent 23.8 million and 13.6 million episodes of antibiotic-treated illness, respectively, among children under five years of age in LMICs each year.

C. Vaccines may reduce the burden of antimicrobial resistance, in part by preventing infections for which treatment often includes the use of antibiotics.

D. By analyzing data from large-scale studies of households, we estimate that pneumococcal conjugate vaccines and live attenuated rotavirus vaccines confer 19.7% (95% confidence interval, 3.4–43.4%) and 11.4% (4.0–18.6%) protection against antibiotic-treated episodes of acute respiratory infection and diarrhea, respectively, in age groups that experience the greatest disease burden attributable to the vaccine-targeted pathogens.

E. However, the effects of vaccination on antibiotic consumption remain poorly understood—especially in low- and middle-income countries (LMICs), where the burden of antimicrobial resistance is greatest.

F. This evidence supports the prioritization of vaccines within the global strategy to combat antimicrobial resistance.

G. Direct protection resulting from the achievement of universal coverage targets for these vaccines could prevent an additional 40.0 million episodes of antibiotic-treated illness.

_____ — _____ — _____ — _____ — _____
_____ — _____ — _____

Task 4

Directions: *(A) The passage below is a section taken from medical research paper. Try to rewrite it into a 4-point abstract with a standard outline. If necessary, add or leave out some unimportant parts. (B) Then select four to six key words for the abstract you have written.*

Members of the US national cross country ski team were found to have significantly lower resting salivary IgA levels than control subjects, and these decreased further after a 50-kilometer race (2-3 hours of exhaustive exercise). To determine whether this decrease in IgA levels might be due to the exercise itself, or might be due to the effects of cold, to the stress of competition, or to a combination of factors, Tomasi and his colleagues conducted a study of competitive cyclists. No differences were found between resting salivary IgA levels in cyclists and controls. However, a 70% decrease in salivary IgA levels was observed immediately after intense endurance exercise. This was not due to the effect of cold, nor to the stress of competition, since they cycled in the laboratory, in a controlled temperature and a non-competitive setting. There was also a significant reduction in NK cell activity. The reduction in IgA and NK cell activity was transitory, returning to pre-exercise level 24 hours after this single bout of severe exercise. The authors conclude that prolonged intense exercise alters parameters of mucosal and natural immunity, and suggest that severe exercise may itself be a form of stress associated with changes in immune reactivity, since the changes occurred in the absence of cold or competition. The authors comment that the suppressive effects of intense exercise may be cumulative, which would explain the low resting IgA levels in their study of skiers who were tested at the end of the competitive season, yet normal levels in the cyclists tested earlier in the season. Low resting serum IgA levels in elite ultra-distance runners rested at the end of the season have also been found.

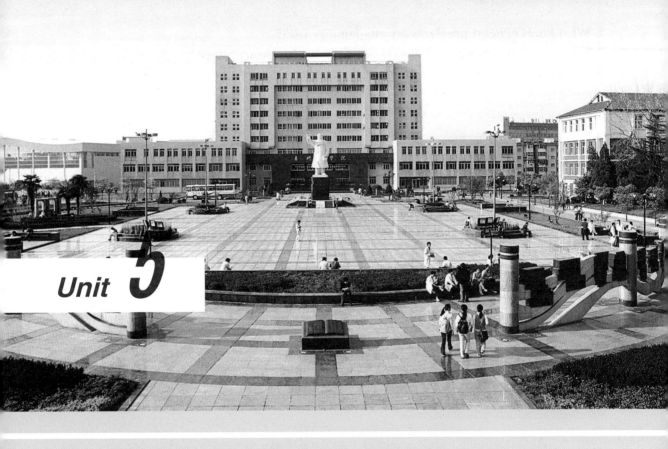

Unit 5

Cardiovascular System I: The Heart and Blood Vessels

√ 听力音频
√ 听力文本
√ 课件资源

Warm-up

1. **What kinds of heart problems are you familiar with?**
2. **What are the common symptoms that may occur in a heart attack?**
3. **What are the possible causes for heart diseases and how can we protect our hearts?**

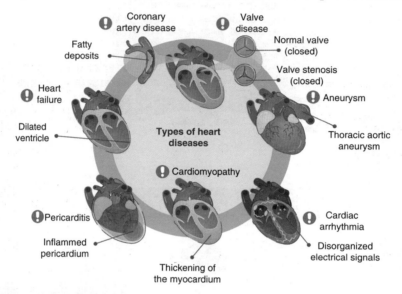

Theme Reading

The Heart and Blood Vessels

In this part, we will learn about the pump that circulates blood throughout the body—the heart. Blood must be constantly pumped through the body's blood vessels so that it can reach body cells and exchange materials with them. To accomplish this, the heart beats about 100,000 times every day, which adds up to 35 million beats in a year and about 2.5 billion times in an average lifetime. Even while you are sleeping, your heart pumps 30 times its own weight (5 L or 5.3 qt) each minute, which amounts to more than 14,000 liters (3,600 gal) of blood in a day and 10 million liters (2.6 million gal) in a year. Because you don't spend all your time sleeping and your heart pumps more vigorously when you are active, the actual blood volume the heart pumps in a single day is even larger. This text explores the structure of the heart and the unique properties that permit it to pump for a lifetime without rest.

Objectives

☆ *Describe location, structure and function of the heart.*
☆ *Describe arteries, veins and capillaries.*

The Heart

Location

The heart is located in the chest, directly above the **diaphragm** in the region of the **thorax** called mediastinum, specifically the middle **mediastinum**. The normal human heart varies with height and weight. The tip (**apex**) of the heart is pointed forward, downward, and toward the left. The (inferior) diaphragmatic surface lies directly on the

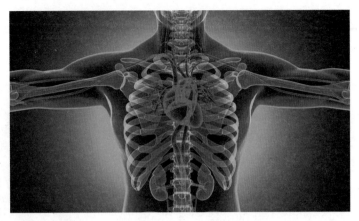

Figure 5-1 Heart location

diaphragm. The heart lies in a double walled fibroserous sac called the **pericardial** sac, which is divided into fibrous pericardium and serous pericardium. The fibrous pericardium envelops the heart and attaches onto the great vessels. The serous pericardium is a closed sac consisting of two layers—a **visceral** layer or **epicardium** forming the outer **lining** of the great vessels and the heart and a **parietal** layer forming an inner lining of the fibrous pericardium. Between these two layers a small amount of fluid exists that is called pericardial fluid, which prevents friction between the heart and the pericardium.

Structure

The wall of the heart is composed of three layers: epicardium, **myocardium** and **endocardium**. The epicardium is the outer lining of the **cardiac** chambers and is formed by the visceral layer of the serous pericardium. The myocardium is the intermediate layer of the heart and is composed of three discernable layers of muscle that are seen predominantly in the left **ventricle** and interventricular **septum** alone and include a subepicardial layer, a middle concentric layer and a subendocardial layer. The rest of the heart is composed mainly of the subepicardial and

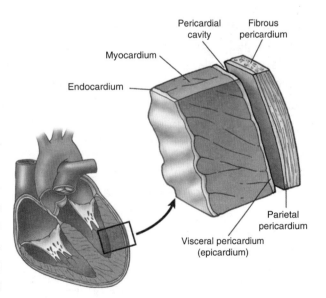

Figure 5-2 Layers of heart wall

subendocardial layers. The myocardium also contains important structures such as excitable nodal tissue and the conducting system. The **endocardium**, the innermost layer of the heart, is formed of the endothelium and subendothelial connective tissue.

Chambers and Valves

The heart is divided into four distinct chambers with muscular walls of different thickness. The left **atrium** (LA) and right atrium (RA) are small, thin-walled chambers located just above the left ventricle (LV) and right ventricle (RV), respectively. The ventricles are larger thick-walled chambers that perform most of the work. The atria receive blood from the venous system and lungs and then contract and eject the blood into the ventricles. The ventricles then pump the blood throughout the body or into the lungs. The heart contains four **valves** and the fibrous skeleton of the heart. The fibrous skeleton, a structure of dense connective tissue that separates the atria from the ventricles, contains the **annuli** of the four valves, membranous septum,

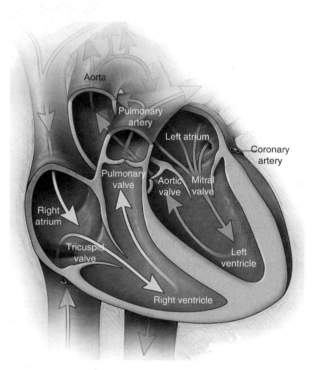

Figure 5-3 Chambers and valves

aortic **intervalvular**, right, and left fibrous trigones. The right trigone and the membranous septum together form the central fibrous body, which is penetrated by the atrioventricular bundle (AV bundle, or bundle of His). The fibrous skeleton functions not only to provide an electrophysiological dissociation of atria and the ventricles, but also provides structural support to the heart. Each of the four valves has a distinctive role in maintaining physiological stability.

The four valves allow blood to flow in only one direction through the heart chambers—from the atria through the ventricles and out the great arteries leaving the heart. The **atrioventricular**, or AV, valves are located between the atrial and ventricular chambers on each side. These valves prevent backflow into the atria when the ventricles contract. The left AV valve—the **bicuspid**, or **mitral**, valve—consists of two **flaps**, or cusps, of endocardium. The right AV valve, the tricuspid valve, has three flaps. When the heart is relaxed and blood is passively filling its chambers, the AV-valve flaps hang limply into the ventricles. As the ventricles contract, they press on the blood in their chambers, and the intraventricular pressure begins to rise. This forces the AV-valve flaps upward, closing the valves. In this manner, the AV valves prevent backflow into the atria when the ventricles are contracting.

The second set of valves, the semilunar valves, guards the bases of the two large arteries leaving the ventricular chambers. Thus, they are known as the pulmonary and aortic semilunar valves. Each semilunar valve has three **leaflets** that fit tightly together when the valves are closed. When the ventricles are contracting and forcing blood out of the heart, the leaflets are forced open and flattened against the walls of the arteries by the tremendous force of rushing blood. When the ventricles relax, the blood begins to flow backward toward the heart, and the leaflets fill with blood, closing the valves. This prevents blood from reentering the heart.

Conduction System of the Heart

The cardiac conduction system consists of highly specialised cells, which are mainly involved in the conduction of **impulses** to the different regions of the myocardium. It has been seen to be composed of three types of morphologically and functionally distinct cells, which include P-cells (Pale/Pacemaker-cells), transitional cells and Purkinje cells. These are important in maintaining the heart's electrical activity in an orderly fashion. The conduction system consists of sinus node, internodal tracts, AV node, AV (His) bundle, right and left bundle branches and Purkinje fibers.

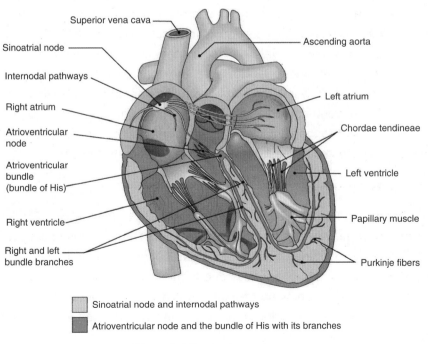

Figure 5-4 Conduction system

Cardiac Cycle

The cardiac cycle is the sequence of events that occurs in one complete beat of the heart. The pumping phase of the cycle, also known as **systole**, occurs when heart muscle contracts. The filling phase, which is known as **diastole**, occurs when heart muscle relaxes. At the beginning of the cardiac cycle, both atria and ventricles are in diastole. During this time, all the chambers of the heart are relaxed and receive blood. The atrioventricular valves are open. Atrial systole follows this phase. During atrial systole, the left and right atria contract at the same time and push blood into the left and right ventricles, respectively. The next phase is ventricular systole. During ventricular systole, the left and right ventricles contract at the same time and pump blood into the **aorta** and pulmonary trunk, respectively. In ventricular systole, the atria are relaxed and receive blood. The atrioventricular valves close immediately after ventricular systole begins to stop blood going back into the atria. However, the semilunar valves are open during this phase to allow the blood to flow into the aorta and pulmonary trunk. Following this phase, the ventricles relax, that is, ventricular diastole occurs. The semilunar valves close to stop the blood from flowing back into the ventricles from the aorta and pulmonary trunk. The atria and ventricles once again are in diastole together and the cycle begins again.

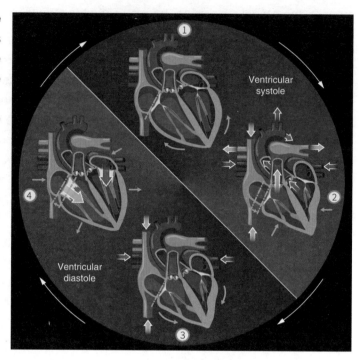

Figure 5-5 Cardiac cycle

Components of the Heartbeat

The adult heart beats around 70 to 80 times a minute at rest. When you listen to your heart with a stethoscope, you can hear your heart beat. The sound is usually described as "lubb-dupp". The "lubb" also known as the first heart sound, is caused by the closure of the atrioventricular valves. The "dupp" sound is due to the closure of the semilunar valves when the ventricles relax (at the beginning of ventricular diastole). Abnormal heart sounds are known as **murmurs**. Murmurs may indicate a problem with the heart valves but many types of murmur are no cause for concern.

Blood Vessels

Artery

Arteries are blood vessels that carry blood away from the heart. This blood is normally oxygenated, exceptions made for the pulmonary and umbilical arteries. The circulatory system is extremely important for sustaining life. Its proper functioning is responsible for the delivery of oxygen and nutrients to all cells, as well as the removal of carbon dioxide and waste products, maintenance of optimum pH, and the mobility of the elements, proteins and cells of the immune system. In developed countries, the two leading causes of death, **myocardial infarction** and **stroke**, each may directly result from an arterial system that has been slowly and progressively compromised by years of deterioration.

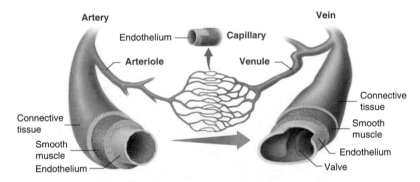

Figure 5-6 Blood vessels

Types of Arteries

The pulmonary arteries carry deoxygenated blood that has just returned from the body to the heart towards the lungs, where carbon dioxide is exchanged for oxygen. Systemic arteries can be subdivided into two types—muscular and elastic—according to the relative compositions of elastic and muscle tissue in their tunica media as well as their size and the makeup of the internal and external elastic **lamina**. The larger arteries (>10 mm diameter) are generally elastic and the smaller ones (0.1—10 mm) tend to be muscular. Systemic **arteries** deliver blood to the arterioles, and then to the capillaries, where nutrients and gasses are exchanged. The aorta is the root systemic artery. It receives blood directly from the left ventricle of the heart via the aortic valve. As the aorta branches, and these arteries branch in turn, they become successively smaller in diameter, down to the arterioles. The arterioles supply capillaries which in turn empty into **venules**. The very first branches off of the aorta are the **coronary** arteries, which supply blood to the heart muscle itself. These are followed by the branches off the aortic arch, namely the **brachiocephalic** artery, the left common **carotid** and the left **subclavian** arteries. Arterioles, the smallest of the true arteries, help regulate blood pressure by the variable contraction of the smooth muscle of their walls and deliver blood to the capillaries.

Vein

In the circulatory system, veins (from the Latin vena) are blood vessels that carry blood towards the heart. Most veins carry deoxygenated blood from the tissues back to the heart; exceptions are the pulmonary and umbilical veins, both of which carry oxygenated blood to the heart.

Veins are classified in a number of ways, including superficial vs. deep, pulmonary vs. systemic and large vs. small. Superficial veins are those whose course is close to the surface of the body, and have no corresponding arteries. Deep veins are deeper in the body and have corresponding arteries. Pulmonary veins are a set of veins that deliver oxygenated blood from the lungs to the heart. Systemic veins drain the tissues of the body and deliver deoxygenated blood to the heart.

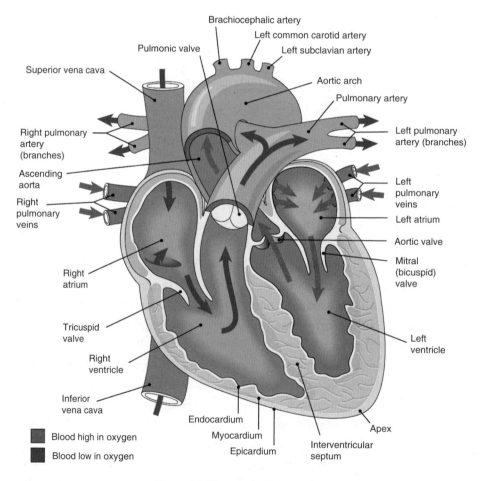

Figure 5-7 Heart and great vessels

Differences between Arteries and Veins

The walls of arteries are usually much thicker than those of veins. This structural difference is related to a difference in function of these two types of vessels. Arteries, which are closer to the pumping action of the heart, must be able to expand as blood is forced into them and then recoil passively as the blood flows off into the circulation during diastole. Their walls must be strong and stretchy enough to take these continuous changes in pressure.

Veins, in contrast, are far from the heart in the circulatory pathway. The pressure in them tends to be low all the time. Thus veins have thinner walls. However, because the blood pressure in veins is usually too low to force the blood back to the heart and because blood returning to the heart often flows against gravity, veins are modified to ensure that the amount of blood returning to the heart equals the amount being pumped out of the heart at any time. The **lumens** of veins tend to be much larger than those of corresponding arteries and the larger veins have valves that prevent backflow of blood.

Capillaries

Capillaries are the smallest of a body's blood vessels and are parts of the microcirculation, where all of the important exchanges happen in the circulatory system. They are only 1 cell thick. These microvessels, measuring 5—10 μm in diameter, connect arterioles and venules and enable the exchange of water, oxygen, carbon dioxide and many other nutrients and waste chemical substances between blood and surrounding tissues. During embryological development, new capillaries are formed by vasculogenesis, the process of blood vessel formation occurring by a de novo production of endothelial cells and their formation into vascular tubes. The term angiogenesis denotes the formation of new capillaries from pre-existing blood vessels.

Vocabulary

annulus [ˈænjʊləs]   (pl. annuli) a toroidal shape

aorta [eɪˈɔːtə]   the main artery through which blood leaves your heart before it flows through the rest of your body

apex [ˈeɪpeks]   the highest or pointed point (of something)

arteriole [ɑːˈtɪərɪəʊl]   one of the small thin-walled arteries that end in capillaries

atrioventricular [ˌeɪtrɪəʊvenˈtrɪkjʊlə]   relating to or affecting the atria and ventricles of the heart

atrium [ˈeɪtrɪəm]   (pl. atria) one of the two upper chambers of the heart

bicuspid [baɪˈkʌspɪd]   having or terminating in two points

brachiocephalic [ˌbrækɪəʊsɪˈfælɪk]   pertaining to the upper limb and the head

cardiac [ˈkɑːdɪæk]   of or relating to the heart

carotid [kəˈrɒtɪd]   of or relating to either of the two major arteries supplying blood to the head and neck

coronary [ˈkɒrənəri]   surrounding like a crown (especially of the blood vessels surrounding the heart)

diaphragm [ˈdaɪəfræm]　muscular partition separating the abdominal and thoracic cavities

diastole [daɪˈæstəli]　the widening of the chambers of the heart between two contractions when the chambers fill with blood

endocardium [ˌendəʊˈkɑːdɪəm]　the membrane that lines the cavities of the heart and forms part of the heart valves

endothelium [ˌendəʊˈθiːlɪəm]　a thin layer of flattened cells that lines the inside of some body cavities

epicardium [ˌepɪˈkɑːdɪəm]　the innermost of the two layers of the pericardium

flap [flæp]　a movable piece of tissue partly connected to the body

impulse [ˈɪmpʌls]　a sudden pushing or driving force

intervalvular [ˌɪntəˈvælvjʊlə]　between the valves

lamina [ˈlæmɪnə]　a thin layer of bone, membrane, or other tissue

leaflet [ˈliːflɪt]　a thin triangular flap of a heart valve

lining [ˈlaɪnɪŋ]　protective covering that protects an inside surface

lumen [ˈluːmɪn]　a cavity or passage in a tubular organ

mediastinum [ˌmiːdɪæsˈtaɪnəm]　the part of the thoracic cavity between the lungs that contains the heart, aorta, esophagus, trachea and thymus

mitral valve [ˈmaɪtrəl]　the cardiac valve between the left atrium and left ventricle, usually having two cusps

murmur [ˈmɜːmə]　an abnormal sound of the heart; sometimes a sign of abnormal function of the heart valves

myocardial infarction [ˌmaɪəʊˈkɑːdɪəl]　destruction of heart tissue resulting from obstruction of the blood supply to the heart muscle

myocardium [ˌmaɪəʊˈkɑːdɪəm]　the middle muscular layer of the heart wall

parietal [pəˈraɪətəl]　of, relating to, or forming the walls or part of the walls of a bodily cavity or similar structure

pericardium [ˌperɪˈkɑːdɪəm]　a double-layered membranous sac that surrounds the heart

septum [ˈseptəm]　a dividing partition between two tissues or cavities

stroke [strəʊk]　the sudden death of brain cells in a localized area due to inadequate blood flow

subclavian [sʌbˈkleɪvɪən]　(of an artery, vein, area, etc.) situated below the clavicle

systole [ˈsɪstəli]　the contraction of the chambers of the heart (especially the ventricles) to drive blood into the aorta and pulmonary artery

thorax [ˈθɔːræks]　the middle region of the body of an arthropod between the head and the abdomen

valve [vælv]　a structure in a hollow organ (like the heart) with a flap to insure one-way flow of fluid through it

ventricle [ˈventrɪkl]　a chamber of the heart that receives blood from an atrium and pumps it to the artery

venule [ˈvenjuːl]　any of the small branches of a vein that receives oxygen-depleted blood from the capillaries and returns it to the heart via the venous system

visceral [ˈvɪsərəl]　relating to or affecting the viscera

Task 1

Directions: *Select the letter of the choice that best completes the statement or answers the question.*

(1) The heart is located in the _____ and serves as the pump of blood circulation.

A. diaphragm   B. epithelium   C. mediastinum   D. metabolism

(2) The heart wall consists of the following parts except _____.

A. pericardium   B. epicardium   C. endocardium   D. myocardium

(3) Among the following, which statement is NOT true about the ventricles?

A. They are larger than the atria.

B. They pump the blood only into the lungs.

C. They receive blood from the atria.

D. Their walls are thicker than those of the atria.

(4) The _____ valve lies between the right atrium and the right ventricle.

A. tricuspid   B. bicuspid   C. semilunar   D. mitral

(5) All the chambers of the heart are relaxed and receive blood during the phase of _____.

A. diastole   B. exhalation   C. systole   D. inhalation

(6) The abnormal sound in the heartbeat is termed _____.

A. diastole   B. flutter   C. systole   D. murmur

(7) The cardiac conduction system consists of all of the components EXCEPT _____.

A. sinus node   B. internodal tracts   C. left ventricle   D. AV bundle

(8) The functions of the circulatory system do NOT include _____.

A. delivery of oxygen and nutrients to all cells

B. removal of carbon dioxide and waste products

C. maintenance of optimum pH

D. fixation of the elements, proteins and cells of the immune system

(9) _____ carry deoxygenated blood that has just returned from the body to the heart towards the lungs.

A. Systemic arteries   B. Pulmonary arteries   C. Muscular arteries   D. Elastic arteries

(10) When measuring BP, the health practitioner is assessing _____.

A. the pressure of blood within the veins

B. the pressure of blood within the arteries

C. the pressure of blood within the heart

D. the pressure of blood within the lungs

Task 2

Directions: *Label the parts of the heart and the vessels.*

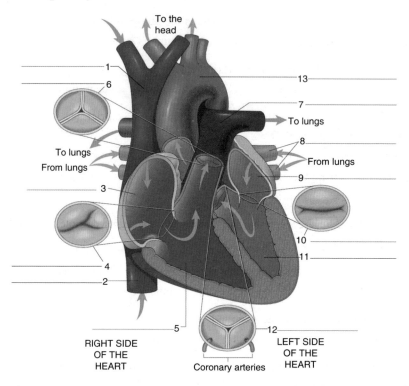

Task 3

Directions: *Fill in the following table based on the text above or relevant information from the Internet and then talk about the heart and blood vessels.*

Structure	Function
(1) aorta	
(2) myocardium	
(3) veins	
(4) pericardium	
(5) atria	
(6) arteries	
(7) valves	
(8) capillaries	
(9) atrioventricular bundle	
(10) ventricles	

Task 4

Directions: *Match each of the following terms in Column A with its definition in Column B.*

A	B
(1) venule	A. the innermost of the two layers of the pericardium
(2) impulse	B. a thin layer of flattened cells that lines the inside of some body cavities
(3) epicardium	C. one of the small thin-walled arteries that end in capillaries
(4) systole	D. any of the small branches of a vein that receives oxygen-depleted blood from the capillaries and returns it to the heart via the venous system
(5) endothelium	E. pertaining to the upper limb and the head
(6) septum	F. the widening of the chambers of the heart between two contractions when the chambers fill with blood
(7) arteriole	G. a dividing partition between two tissues or cavities
(8) carotid	H. a sudden pushing or driving force
(9) brachiocephalic	I. the contraction of the chambers of the heart (especially the ventricles) to drive blood into the aorta and pulmonary artery
(10) diastole	J. of or relating to either of the two major arteries supplying blood to the head and neck

Medical Terminology

Roots	Terminology	Term Analysis	Definition
heart			
cardi(o) ['kɑ:dɪəʊ]	cardialgia [ˌkɑ:dɪ'ældʒɪə] cardiodynia [ˌkɑ:dɪəʊ'dɪnɪə] cardiology [ˌkɑ:dɪ'ɒlədʒi]	-algia=pain	
coron(o) ['kɒrənəʊ]	coronary ['kɒrənəri] coronavirus [kəˌrəʊnə'vaɪərəs]	-ary=pertaining to	
aorta			
aort(o) [eɪ'ɔ:təʊ]	aortic [eɪ'ɔ:tɪk] aortogram [eɪ'ɔ:təgræm]	-ic=pertaining to	
atrium			
atri(o) ['eɪtrɪəʊ]	transatrial [træns'eɪtrɪəl] atriomegaly [ˌeɪtrɪəʊ'megli]	trans-=across, through	

(to be continued)

ventricle			
ventricul(o) [venˈtrɪkjʊləʊ]	supraventricular [ˌsjuːprəvenˈtrɪkjʊlə] ventriculoscope [venˈtrɪkjʊləskəʊp]	supra-=above, upper	
valve			
valv(o) [ˈvælvəʊ] valvul(o) [ˈvælvjʊləʊ]	valvoplasty [ˈvælvəplæsti] valvulotomy [ˌvælvjʊˈlɒtəmi] valvulitis [ˌvælvjʊˈlaɪtɪs]	-tomy=incision, cutting into	
vessel			
angi(o) [ˈændʒɪəʊ]	angiofibroma [ˌændʒɪəʊfaɪˈbrəʊmə] angiostenosis [ˌændʒɪəʊstɪˈnəʊsɪs]	fibro=fiber	
vas(o) [ˈvæsəʊ] vascul(o) [ˈvæskjʊləʊ]	vasography [væˈsɒgrəfi] vasospasm [ˈvæsəʊspæzəm] vasculitis [ˌvæskjʊˈlaɪtɪs] vasculopathy [ˌvæskjʊˈlɒpəθi]		
artery			
arteri(o) [ɑːˈtɪərɪəʊ]	arteritis [ˌɑːtəˈraɪtɪs] arteralgia [ˌɑːtəˈrældʒɪə] arteriomalacia [ɑːˌtɪərɪəʊməˈleɪʃɪə] arterionecrosis [ɑːˌtɪərɪəʊneˈkrəʊsɪs]	-malacia=softening	
arteriole			
arteriol/o [ɑːˌtɪərɪˈəʊləʊ]	arteriolar [ɑːˌtɪərɪˈəʊlə] arteriolosclerosis [ɑːˌtɪərɪˌəʊləʊsklɪəˈrəʊsɪs]	-sclerosis=hardening	
vein			
phleb(o) [ˈflebəʊ]	endophlebitis [ˌendəʊflɪˈbaɪtɪs] phleborrhagia [ˌflebəʊˈreɪdʒɪə]	-rrhagia=bursting forth (of blood)	

(to be continued)

ven(o) [ˈviːnəʊ] ven(i) [ˈveni]	intravenous [ˌɪntrəˈviːnəs] venoclysis [viːˈnɒklɪsɪs] venipuncture [ˈvenɪˌpʌŋktʃə] venisuture [ˈvenɪsjuːtʃə]		
venule			
venul(o) [ˈvenjʊləʊ]	venulitis [ˌvenjʊˈlaɪtɪs]		
chest			
steth(o) [ˈsteθəʊ]	stethoscope [ˈsteθəskəʊp] stethomyitis [ˌsteθəʊmaɪˈaɪtɪs]		
thorac(o) [ˈθɔːrəkəʊ]	thoracostenosis [ˌθɔːrəkəʊstɪˈnəʊsɪs] thoracostomy [ˌθɔːrəˈkɒstəmi]	-stenosis=narrowing; strirction	

Vocabulary Study

Task 1

Directions: *Match each of the following terms with its definition and underline the strong part of each word where there are two or more syllables.*

(1) arteriolar	A. surgical formation of an opening into the chest cavity
(2) arteritis	B. within or administered into a vein
(3) intravenous	C. inflammation of an artery
(4) thoracostomy	D. puncture of a vein through the skin in order to withdraw blood
(5) venipuncture	E. pertaining to an arteriole or the arterioles

(6) phleborrhagia	A. incision into a stenosed cardiac valve to relieve the obstruction
(7) stethomyitis	B. bleeding from a vein
(8) transatrial	C. performed through the atrium
(9) vasospasm	D. inflammation of the muscles of the chest wall
(10) valvulotomy	E. a sudden constriction of a blood vessel

Task 2

Directions: *Fill in the blanks with appropriate words for body parts.*

(1) A person with arteralgia has a pain in the _____.

(2) Ventriculoscope refers to the instrument used to examine the _____.

(3) A person with coronary diseases has some diseases affecting the _____ and coronary _____.

(4) A person with angiostenosis has a narrowing of one or more _____.

(5) An aortogram is an X-ray film or record of the _____.

(6) A person who has valvulitis has an inflammation of the _____.

(7) Venotomy is an incision of a _____ for the removal or withdrawal of blood.

(8) Cardiology is the study of the _____ and its diseases.

(9) Arteriolosclerosis means the hardening and thickening of the walls of _____.

(10) A person who has atriomegaly has an enlargement of the _____.

Task 3

Directions: *Write a word for each of the following definitions using the word parts provided.*

-ic	cardi(o)	ventricul(o)	aort(o)	phleb(o)
-scope	valvul(o)	-logy	-itis	-tomy

(1) pertaining to the aorta _____

(2) the study of the heart and its diseases _____

(3) inflammation of the vein _____

(4) instrument used to view and examine the ventricle _____

(5) incision of a heart valve _____

arter(o)	-megaly	angi(o)	-sclerosis	-pathy
atri(o)	-stenosis	-algia	arteri(o)	vascul(o)

(6) disease of the blood vessels _____

(7) hardening and thickening of the arteries _____

(8) enlargement of the atrium of the heart _____

(9) pain in the artery _____

(10) narrowing of one or more blood vessels _____

| valv(o) | arteri(o) | -plasty | ven(o) | -graphy |
| thorac(o) | aort(o) | -ostomy | -malacia | -clysis |

(11) surgical formation of an opening into the chest cavity _____

(12) surgical repair of the valve _____

(13) softening of the arteries _____

(14) injection of fluid into a vein _____

(15) examination of the aorta using x-rays _____

Case Study 5-1

Infective Endocarditis

E.F. is a 72-year-old man who comes to the clinic with "flulike" symptoms. He has a history of hypertension, past MRSA infection, and a recently implanted pacemaker. E.F. has petechiae in the conjunctivae and splinter hemorrhages in his nail beds. His blood pressure is 138/64, heart rate 80, respiratory rate 18, and temperature 99.5° F (37.5° C). Physical examination revealed a pansystolic murmur over the apex and left lower sternal border. Transthoracic echocardiography revealed a vegetation with size of 0.9 cm over the anterior leaflet of mitral valve, and moderate mitral regurgitation. However, the cardiac systolic and diastolic functions were normal. The health care provider suspects infective endocarditis, an infection of the endocardium, which is often difficult to recognize and therefore easily missed in the emergency department.

E.F. is sent to the hospital for further workup and treatment and his blood culture results are positive for Staphylococcus aureus. E.F. is started on IV antibiotics and seems to be resting comfortably. He occasionally requests PRN drugs for "achiness" and continues to have a low-grade fever. He is not demonstrating any symptoms of heart failure at this time. E.F. has completed a week of IV antibiotic therapy in the hospital setting. He is afebrile and feeling better. Social service has arranged home IV antibiotic therapy in anticipation of discharge to home.

Task 4

Directions: Select the best answer to the question or the statement based on the information provided in the case of infective endocarditis.

(1) The term "hypertension" means _____.

    A. abnormally low blood pressure   B. abnormally high blood pressure

    C. abnormally low blood sugar   D. abnormally high blood sugar

(2) Which of the following is the function of a pacemaker?

    A. To help control your heartbeat.

    B. To treat a slow heartbeat after a heart attack or surgery.

    C. To help your heart beat more regularly.

    D. All of the above.

(3) The pansystolic murmur extends through _____.

    A. the first half of the systolic interval   B. the second half of the systolic interval

    C. the entire systolic interval   D. the middle of the systolic interval

(4) The term "transthoracic" means across or through the _____.

    A. chest wall   B. throat   C. diaphragm   D. mediastinum

(5) The term "echocardiography" refers to _____.

    A. the instrument to examine the heart

    B. examination of the heart using ultrasound techniques

    C. the film of the heart produced after the examination

    D. the person who does the examination of the heart

(6) Which of the following words has the meaning of "backflow of blood through a defective heart valve"?

    A. Eructation.   B. Flatulence.   C. Regurgitation.   D. Vegetation.

(7) Diastolic pressure refers to the blood pressure when _____.

    A. the heart muscle relaxes   B. the heart muscle convulses

    C. the heart muscle contracts   D. the heart muscle constricts

(8) Endocarditis may occur _____.

    A. outside the heart   B. within the heart

    C. over the heart   D. under the heart

(9) IV antibiotics are injected into the patient _____.

    A. under the skin   B. through an artery

    C. within a capillary   D. through or within a vein

(10) What will E.F. do after completing a week of antibiotic therapy in the hospital?

    A. He will receive another round of antibiotic therapy in the community.

    B. He will go to the nursing home for total recovery.

    C. He will go back home and still receive antibiotic therapy for some time.

    D. He will go to live in the social service center.

Case Study 5-2

Mitral Valve Replacement Operative Report

A.L. was diagnosed with mitral prolapse with regurgitation and was transferred to the operating room, placed in a supine position, and given general endotracheal anesthesia. Her pericardium was entered longitudinally through a median sternotomy. The surgeon found that her heart was enlarged with a dilated right ventricle. The left atrium was dilated. Preoperative transesophageal echocardiogram revealed severe mitral regurgitation with severe posterior and anterior prolapse. Extracorporeal circulation was established. The aorta was cross-clamped, and cardioplegic solution (to stop the heartbeat) was given into the aortic root intermittently for myocardial protection.

The left atrium was entered via the interatrial groove on the right, exposing the mitral valve. The middle scallop of the posterior leaflet was resected. The remaining leaflets were removed to the areas of the commissures and preserved for the sliding plasty. The elongated chordae were shortened. The surgeon slid the posterior leaflet across the midline and sutured it in place. A No. 30 annuloplasty ring was sutured in place with interrupted No. 2-0 Dacron suture. The valve was tested by inflating the ventricle with NSS and proved to be competent. The left atrium was closed with continuous No. 4-0 Prolene suture. Air was removed from the heart. The cross-clamp was removed. Cardiac action resumed with normal sinus rhythm. After a period of cardiac recovery and attainment of normothermia, cardiopulmonary bypass was discontinued.

Protamine was given to counteract the heparin. Pacer wires were placed in the right atrium and ventricle. Silicone catheters were placed in the pleural and substernal spaces. The sternum and soft tissue wound was closed. A. L. recovered from her surgery and was discharged 6 days later.

Task 5

Directions: *Write a word or phrase from the case study that means the same as each of the following.*

(1) the double-layered membranous sac that completely envelops the heart _____

(2) incision into the breastbone _____

(3) a graphical image of the heart produced by ultrasound technique _____

(4) backflow of blood through a defective heart valve _____

(5) falling down of an organ or part from its normal position _____

(6) pertaining to the muscular tissue of the heart _____

(7) between the upper chambers of the heart _____

(8) Reconstruction of the ring (or annulus) of a cardiac valve _____

(9) a condition of normal body temperature _____

(10) pertaining to or affecting both the heart and the lungs and their functions _____

Medical Term Extension

Diagnostic Equipment

Diagnostic medical equipment and supplies help clinicians to measure and observe various aspects of a patient's health so that they can form a diagnosis. Once a diagnosis is made, the clinician can then prescribe an appropriate treatment plan. Diagnostic medical equipment is found in outpatient care centers for adult and pediatrics, in emergency rooms, as well as inpatient hospital rooms and intensive care units.

The following list is not exhaustive, but it provides an overview of some of the most commonly used diagnostic tools.

Thermometer

Thermometers are used in all areas and levels of care, from routine physical exams to emergency department triage to inpatient care. There are now electronic thermometers that shorten the time necessary to measure a patient's temperature. The electronic ones can be set for the specific part of the body being measured, such as the mouth, the armpit, the rectum, or the ear.

Stethoscopes

Stethoscopes are probably the most recognizable of all medical diagnostic tools. They are used to listen to heart sounds, the lungs, and even blood flow in the arteries and veins. Stethoscopes are also used along with a sphygmomanometer to measure blood pressure.

Electronic stethoscopes improve sound quality when listening to the low-pitched heart sounds and the high-pitched pulmonary sounds. They can be connected to a computer to record and save the sounds. They can be hooked up to distributors that allow multiple people to listen to adjoining stethoscopes. This last feature is important when training interns, residents, and fellows.

Sphygmomanometers

High blood pressure has been linked to several diseases. There are a few products that are used to measure blood pressure.

Manual sphygmomanometers are considered the most reliable. Mercury manometers don't require routine calibration and therefore are used in high-risk scenarios.

Aneroid sphygmomanometers are a little less reliable because they can lose their calibration when bumped, which can be a common occurrence in healthcare settings. Wall-mounted styles can reduce this possibility, but should still have calibration checks to be sure. The aneroid style is easily identified as a mechanical unit with a dial for the readings, as well as a bulb and air valve.

Digital finger blood pressure monitors are the smallest and most portable. While easy to operate, they are a bit less accurate.

Digital sphygmomanometers, like the digital finger blood pressure monitors, are also electronic. They can be inflated either manually or automatically. They are easy to use but derive blood pressure in an indirect way. Digital units measure mean arterial pressure, which basically translates into an average of the systolic and diastolic pressure. The digital sphygmomanometer then must derive what the systolic and diastolic readings would be. These are helpful in noisy areas where the manual mercury manometers would prove ineffective because of the need for the clinician to hear the Korotkoff sounds.

Electrocardiographs

Electrocardiographs measure the electrical activity of the heart.

During this examination, heart rate can be recorded, as well as the regularity of the beats. These are two key indicators of any issues in the heart. Physicians can even read an electrocardiograph to determine the size and position of each heart chamber. And finally, a major use for the electrocardiograph is to diagnose damage to the heart and the impact and efficacy of drug treatment or device implant.

Ophthalmoscopes

Ophthalmoscopes are handheld tools that allow a physician to see into the fundus of a patient's eye. This type of diagnostic tool is commonly used in physical or outpatient exams. There are two types of ophthalmoscopes.

Direct ophthalmoscopes produce an upright image of approximately 15 times magnification. These tools are held as close to the patient's eye as possible.

Indirect ophthalmoscopes produce an inverted image of 2 to 5 times magnification. Indirect ophthalmoscopes are held 24 to 30 inches from the patient's eye. Indirects also have a more powerful light so they are more effective than directs when used in patients with cataracts.

Otoscopes

Otoscopes are handheld devices that allow physicians to look into the ear canal and view the tympanic membrane through the magnification lens.

The head of the otoscope also has a light. The light, together with the magnifying lens, makes it possible to view the outer and middle ear. The portion that the physician inserts into the ear canal is called the disposable speculum. Disposable specula are stored in a dispenser in the exam room so that a new, clean one can be attached to the otoscopes for each patient.

Task 6

Directions: *Name the following items in English.*

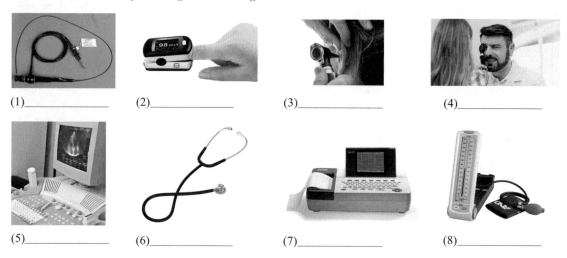

(1)_____ (2)_____ (3)_____ (4)_____

(5)_____ (6)_____ (7)_____ (8)_____

Task 7

Directions: *Read the following article. Then, think about for what condition the diagnostic equipment below is used.*

Hewlett Medical
AN INDUSTRY LEADER

DIAGNOSTIC

EQUIPMENT

When it comes to diagnostic equipment, you can trust Hewlett Medical. Our products assist medical professionals and patients in a variety of settings. Our equipment creates visual presentations of things you couldn't see otherwise, both large and small. For example, our ECG and EEG devices show healthcare professionals what the heart and brain are doing. And our spectrophotometers help test nucleic acids.

We also manufacture point-of-care testing devices. Our glucose monitors assist diabetics around the world. Our oximeters are standard equipment in many hospitals.

But Hewlett Medical is always pushing forward. We're combining biosensors to provide more information in less time. Our goal is to combine thermal sensors, mechanical sensors, optical sensors and electrical sensors into a single device. Someday, we hope a single scan will tell medical professionals everything they need to know.

Writing

Medical Abstract (II)

By reading an abstract, the reader can understand the broad content, results and conclusions without needing to read the whole paper. However, different SCI journal has different requirements for abstract writing, which are detailed in "Instructions to Authors" or "Guideline for Authors". The author should write his/her abstract according to the writing requirements of the journal, or modify the abstract to meet the requirements of the target journal.

Writing Requirements of Different Journals for Abstracts

NEJM for Abstract

Provide an abstract of not more than 250 words. It should consist of four paragraphs, labelled Background, Methods, Results and Conclusion. They should briefly describe, respectively the problem being addressed in the study, how the study was performed, the salient results, and what the author conclude from the others.

It can be seen that *NEJM* requires authors to put forward structured abstracts.

Science for Abstract

In the Instructions to Authors, *Science* details its writing requirements for the abstract as:

> Abstracts explain to the general reader why the research was done and why the results are important. They should start with some brief BACKGROUND information: a sentence giving a broad introduction to the field comprehensible to the general reader, and then a sentence of more detailed background specific to your study. This should be followed by the RESULTS, or if the paper is more methods/technique oriented, an explanation of OBJECTIVES/METHODS and then the RESULTS. The final sentence should outline the main CONCLUSION of the study, in terms that will be comprehensible to all our readers. The abstract should be 125 words or less.

In the Instructions to Authors of *Science*, it is suggested that *Science* usually requires non-structured abstracts.

Internal Medicine Journal for Abstract

Internal Medicine Journal makes the following abstract requirements in its author guideline:

> Each manuscript should carry a structured abstract of no more than 250 words presented in the following form. Background: brief statement of relevant work or clinical situation, and hypothesis, if applicable. Aims: brief statement of the overall aim. Methods: laboratory or other techniques used, including statistical analysis. Outcome measures clearly stated. Results: statistically significant results and relevant negative data cited. Conclusions: referable to the aims of the study and may include suggestions for future action.

Attributes of a Good Abstract

A well-written abstract is characterized by the four criteria, viz. it should be complete, concise, clear and cohesive.

A good abstract should be complete. It should be a stand-alone document and cover all the major parts of the research in addition to bringing out its novelty.

A good abstract should be crisp and free from excessive wordiness or unnecessary information. For example, "X stimulates Y" will be a better choice of words than "X produces a stimulatory effect on Y". A good abstract should avoid too much background information. You should refrain from using empty phrases like "It was interesting to note that ....". Cliché statements like "More research is needed" should be avoided. If there are implications, then you must state them clearly.

The abstract should be clear, i.e., readable, well-organized, and not too jargon-laden. Abstract written in active voice provides greater clarity. So, we may write "We conclude that…" instead of "It was concluded that…." The findings of your research should not be discussed in the abstract, and any discussion should only be done in the main text of your research paper. The abstract should be free of figures, diagrams, tables, or images. The abstract should not contain any references/citations. Avoid use of abbreviations or acronyms.

A well written abstract should be cohesive and the text should flow smoothly between the parts. The abstract must follow the chronological order of sections in your main research paper ensuring a smooth transition. It must read like a story. A direct cohesiveness needs to be maintained between objectives, main outcome measures, results and conclusion.

Before you finally submit your abstract check it for consistency; a mismatch between the abstract and main text may raise doubts on authenticity of your results. Check if the abstract meets the guidelines to authors in terms of format, word count, etc.

Choosing of the Keywords

The keywords you choose are important as these are used for indexing purposes. Keywords are listed below the abstract text. It is important to not duplicate the "keywords" and "words used in the main title" as both enable accession and hence citation of your research work. Using the right keywords will speed up the Internet retrieval of your work. In order to determine the keywords, read through your paper and list the terms, phrases and abbreviations used frequently. Try to include variants of a term/phrase already used in your title as keywords; e.g., sepsis and septicemia, renal and kidney, tumor and cancer. Now refer to an indexing standard like the Medical Subject Headings (MeSH) database of the US National Library of Medicine. Check if these terms are listed therein. The MeSH uses two tools to determine keywords:

• MeSH on demand
available from https://www.nlm.nih.gov/mesh/MeSHOnDemand.html
• MeSH browser

available from https://www.nlm.nih.gov/mesh/ MBrowser.html

MeSH on demand is a simple tool, which automatically deciphers the keywords from text such as an abstract or summary. MeSH Browser is a tool, which allows for searches of MeSH terms, text-word searches of the Annotation and Scope Note, and searches of various fields for chemicals. Another way to identify keywords is to search similar research work from PubMed and then ascertain the MeSH headings assigned to them. The keywords are not necessarily single words but may be two words. For example, "breast cancer" is listed as keywords in MeSH.

Before you finally submit your article, check if the keywords are appropriate. Type the keywords into the search engine and see if the search results resemble your research work.

Task 1

Directions: *Sort out the relevant information in an abstract under different moves.*

Moves or key elements in the research paper		
Move	Key elements	Functions / contents/ tense
Move 1	Introduction/Background	introduces the background, present situation, problems, etc., usually written in the present tense.
Move 2	Purpose	states the premise, purpose, problem, task, or thesis of the research, usually written in the past tense.
Move 3	Methods	states the principles, objects, population, location, materials, technology, methods or procedures of the research, usually written in the past tense.
Move 4	Results	state the results, such as the data, effects or properties of the research, usually written in the past tense.
Move 5	Conclusion/Implications	gives comparison or application of the results, or raises questions, recommendations or predictions on the basis of the results, usually written in the present tense.

(1) _____ In contrast with previous research, our study found that lorazepam was as effective as diazepam on all outcome measures in patients with uncomplicated alcohol withdrawal. A likely explanation is that we used higher doses of lorazepam, and a longer treatment duration with a slower taper. We conclude that lorazepam can and should be preferred over diazepam in alcoholics with known or suspected liver disease.

(2) _____ The antidepressant efficacy of desvenlafaxine (DV) has been established in 8-week, randomized controlled trials. The present study examined the continued efficacy of DV across 6 months of maintenance treatment.

(3) _____ The putative hypnotic benefits of melatonin have not been examined inpatients with insomnia arising from medical causes.

(4) _____ At the 7-year follow-up, 52,500 (74.9%) mother-child pairs were re-examined. Attention-deficit hyperactivity disorder (ADHD) was identified in 945 (1.8%) children. Maternal

[odds ratio (OR), 5.2; 95% confidenceinterval (CI),3.4—9.1] and paternal (OR, 3.3; 95% CI, 2.0—5.8) ADHD were each associated with increased risk of ADHD in the offspring. ADHD was more common in male than in female children (OR, 4.8; 95% CI, 2.6—8.5). Maternal age, prematurity, low birth weight, fetal distress, and neonatal asphyxia were not associated with an increased 7-year risk of ADHD. After adjusting for maternal ADHD, intranatal exposure to psychotropic medication did not predict the 7-year risk of ADHD (OR, 1.2; 95% CI, .6—2.8).

(5) _____ Consecutive consenting male inpatients in moderately severe, uncomplicated alcohol withdrawal at screening were randomized to receive either lorazepam(8 mg/day; n=50) or chlordiazepoxide (80 mg/day; n=50) with dosing down-titrated to zero in a fixed-dose schedule across 8 treatment days.

(6) _____ The 9.3% prevalence of bipolar spectrum disorders in students at an arts university is substantially higher than general population estimates. These findings strengthen the oft-expressed hypothesis linking creativity with affective psychopathology.

Task 2

Directions: *Some journals use different headings to those in the BMJ. Match the headings (1—5) to the corresponding BMJ headings (a—e).*

> (1) Findings   a. Introduction
> (2) Purpose   b. Objective
> (3) Background   c. Subjects
> (4) Interpretation   d. Results
> (5) Participants   e. Conclusion

Task 3

Directions: *Fill in the blanks with proper words as required by the context.*

(1) Previous clinical studies have _____（证实）that injectable gold salts and the oral gold compound, auranofin, possess significant steroid-sparing effects in the treatment of asthma. The objectives of this investigation were to _____（确定）whether auranofin could reduce oral corticosteroid requirements.

(2) Objective: To _____（评价）the prevalence of hepatitis C virus (HCV) infection in diabetic patients and to _____（了解）the influence of several epidemiological and clinical factors on HCV infection.

(3) To _____（报告）three cases of idiopathic retroperitoneal fibrosis（IRF, 突发性腹膜后纤维化）_____（诊断）by the fine needle aspiration (FNA) biopsy and _____（证实）by histological examination. _____（就我们所知），this is the first report on the FNA findings in IRF.

(4) Carotid endarterectomy is usually delayed for two months following an acute stroke, but the stroke may _____（发展）or a further stroke may _____（发生）. A _____（随机）pilot study of urgent carotid surgery for acute stroke was _____（进行）to _____（评价）the

feasibility of a definitive multicenter trial.

(5) During the 1980s, the frequency of nosocomial candidiasis（医院念珠病）increased _____（很大）. This trend has _____（持续到）the 1990s, and Candida species _____（仍旧是）a major cause of nosocomial infections. Although Candida albicans（白色念珠菌）remains the most frequent cause of fungemia and hematogenously disseminated candidiasis, a number of reports have _____（证实）infections caused by other candida species. Many of these infections _____（产生于）an endogenous _____（源）, and their frequency is influenced by the patient population, the various treatment _____（方案）, and the antibodies or other supportive care measures employed at specific institutions.

(6) Patients who _____（做）genetic tests for familial adenomatous polyposis often _____（做）inadequate counseling and would have been given incorrectly interpreted results. _____（医生）should be prepared to offer genetic counseling if they order genetic tests.

(7) This article _____（提出）a method for _____（评估）HIV risk in low-HIV-prevalent populations.

(8) We _____（使用）1 mg glucagons intravenously to 5 healthy _____（人群）taking 300 mg allopurinol orally, and determined plasma _____（浓度）and urinary excretion of oxypurinol and purine bases.

(9) A _____（总数）of 337 persons are living in the city of Lund and were born in 1908. Participation _____（率）was 67%. Abnormal findings were _____（进一步）examined and treated.

(10) Efficacy was _____（鉴定）in 119 patients who completed the full protocol, and the results were similar to those obtained in 186 patients who _____（符合）the validity criteria for analysis.

Task 4

Directions: *A well-written abstract should be complete, concise, clear and cohesive. Consider the following examples and decide which version is better than the other. Then think about any other attributes of a well-written abstract.*

Example 1

"Response rates differed significantly between hypertensive and non-hypertensive children."
"The response rate was higher in non-hypertensive than in hypertensive children (50% vs 20%, respectively; P<0.01)."

Example 2

"The time for resolution of diarrhea, and the recovery in terms of resolution of diarrhea and need for hospitalization was similar in the probiotic and placebo groups."
"The median time for resolution of diarrhea was 54 hours in both the probiotic and the placebo group. Recovery in the probiotic group was marginally better but not statistically significant for resolution (hazard ratio = 0.91, 95% CI 0.60—1.31), rehydration (hazard ratio=0.91, 95% CI 0.64—1.39) and hospitalization (hazard ratio = 0.94, 95% CI 0.67—1.34)."

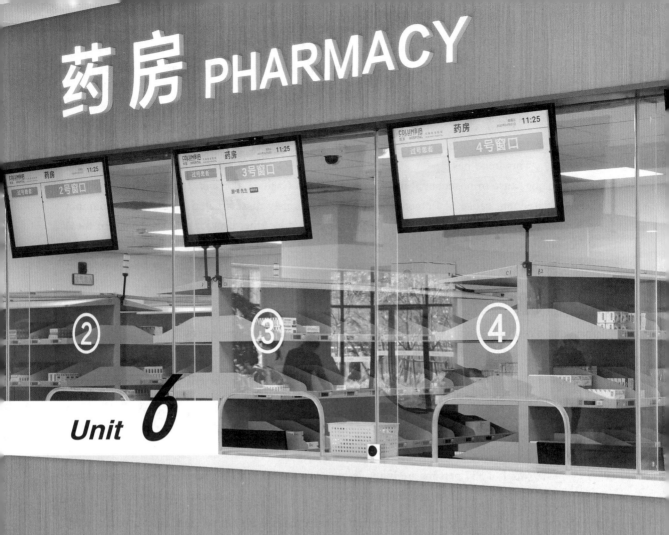

Unit *6*

Cardiovascular System II: The Blood and Blood Circulation

√ 听力音频
√ 听力文本
√ 课件资源

Warm-up

1. What do you know about World Blood Donor Day?

2. Why are blood donations needed all over the world?

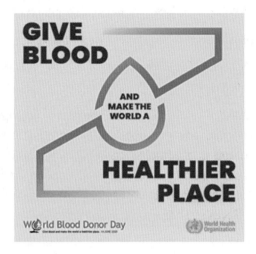

Theme Reading

The Blood and Blood Circulation

For all of its similarities in origin, composition and functions, blood is as unique from one person to another as are skin, bone and hair. Long before modern medicine, blood was viewed as magical, because when it drained from the body, life departed as well. Health-care professionals routinely examine and analyse its differences through various blood tests when trying to determine the cause of different diseases. In this part, we consider the composition and function of this life-sustaining fluid and its circulation.

Objectives

☆ *Describe the composition and volume of whole blood.*

☆ *Describe the composition of plasma.*

☆ *List the cell types making up the formed elements and describe the major functions of each type.*

☆ *Describe the two circuits of blood circulation.*

☆ *Define pulse and blood pressure.*

Physical Characteristics and Volume

Blood is a sticky opaque fluid with a characteristic metallic taste. Depending on the amount of oxygen it is carrying, the color of blood varies from scarlet (oxygen-rich) to a dull red (oxygen-poor). Blood is heavier than water and about five times thicker, or more **viscous**, largely because of its formed elements. Blood is slightly **alkaline**, with a pH between 7.35 and 7.45. Its temperature (38℃ or 100.4 ℉) is always slightly higher than body temperature.

Blood accounts for approximately 8 % of body weight and its volume in healthy men is 5 to 6 liters or about 6 quarts.

Components

Blood is unique: it is the only fluid tissue in the body. Although blood appears to be a thick and homogeneous liquid, the microscope reveals that it has both solid and liquid components. Essentially, blood is a complex connective tissue in which living blood cells, the formed elements, are suspended in a nonliving fluid matrix called **plasma**. The collagen and **elastin** fibers typical of other connective tissues are absent from blood, but dissolved proteins become visible as **fibrin** strands during blood clotting.

If a sample of blood is spun in a centrifuge, the formed elements, being heavier, are packed down by centrifugal force and the plasma rises to the top. Most of the reddish mass at the bottom of the tube is **erythrocyte**, or red blood cells, the formed elements that function in oxygen transport. There is a thin, whitish layer called the buffy coat at the junction between the erythrocytes and the plasma. This layer contains the remaining formed elements, **leukocytes**, the white blood cells that act in various ways to protect the body, and **platelets**, cell fragments that help stop bleeding. Erythrocytes normally account for about 45% of the total volume of a blood sample, a percentage known as the **hematocrit**. White blood cells and platelets contribute less than 1 %, and plasma makes up most of the remaining 55 % of whole blood.

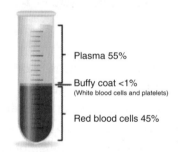

Figure 6-1 Composition of whole blood

Plasma

Plasma, which is approximately 90% water, is the liquid part of the blood. Over 100 different substances are dissolved in this straw-colored fluid. Examples of dissolved substances include **nutrients**, salts, respiratory gases, **hormones**, plasma proteins and various wastes and products of cell metabolism.

The composition of plasma varies continuously as cells remove or add substances to the blood. Assuming a healthy diet, however, the composition of plasma is kept relatively constant by various **homeostatic** mechanisms of the body. For example, when blood proteins drop to undesirable levels, the liver is stimulated to make more proteins, and when the blood starts to become too acid or too basic, both the respiratory system and the kidneys are called into action to restore it to its normal.

Formed Elements

If you observe a stained smear of human blood under a light microscope, you will see disc-shaped red blood cells, a variety of gaudily stained spherical white blood cells, and some scattered platelets that look like debris. However, erythrocytes vastly outnumber the other types of formed elements.

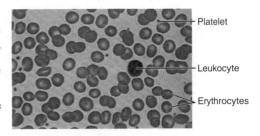

Figure 6-2 Blood cells

Erythrocytes, or red blood cells (RBCs), function primarily to ferry oxygen in blood to all cells of the body. RBCs differ from other blood cells because they are **anucleate**; that is, they lack a nucleus. They also contain very few **organelles**. In fact, mature RBCs circulating in the blood are literally "bags" of **hemoglobin** molecules. Hemoglobin (Hb), an iron-bearing protein, transports the bulk of the oxygen that is carried in the blood. (It also binds with a small amount of carbon dioxide.) RBCs are small, flexible cells shaped like biconcave discs—flattened discs with depressed centers on both sides. Because of their thinner centers, they look like miniature doughnuts when viewed with a microscope. RBCs outnumber white blood cells by about 1,000:1 and are the major factors contributing to blood **viscosity**. Although the numbers of RBCs in the circulation do vary, there are normally about 5 million cells per cubic millimeter of blood.

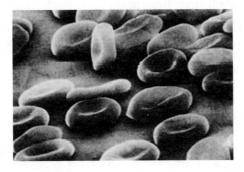

Figure 6-3 Erythrocytes

Although leukocytes, or white blood cells (WBCs), are far less numerous than red blood cells, they are crucial to body defense against diseases. On average, there are 4,000 to 11,000 WBC/mm^3, and they account for less than 1 % of total blood volume. White blood cells are the only complete cells in blood; that is, they contain nuclei and the usual organelles. Leukocytes form a protective, movable army that helps defend the body against damage by bacteria, viruses, parasites and tumor cells. As such, they have some very special characteristics. Red blood cells are confined to the blood stream and carry out their functions in the blood. White blood cells, by contrast, are able to slip into and out of the blood vessels—a process called **diapedesis**. In addition, WBCs can locate areas of tissue damage and infection in the body by responding to certain chemicals that diffuse from the damaged cells. Whenever WBCs mobilize for action, the body speeds up their production, and as many as twice the normal numbers of WBCs may appear in the blood within a few hours. WBCs are classified into two major groups—**granulocytes** and **agranulocytes**—depending on whether or not they contain visible granules in their **cytoplasm**.

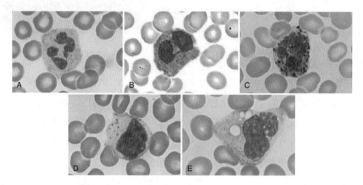

Figure 6-4 Leukocytes
A. Neutrophil B. Eosinophil C. Basophil D. Lymphocyte E. Monocyte

Platelets are not cells in the strict sense. They are fragments of bizarre **multinucleate** cells called **megakaryocytes**, which pinch off thousands of anucleate platelet "pieces" that quickly seal themselves off from the surrounding fluids. The platelets appear as darkly staining, irregularly shaped bodies scattered among the other blood cells. The normal platelet count in blood is about $300,000/mm^3$.

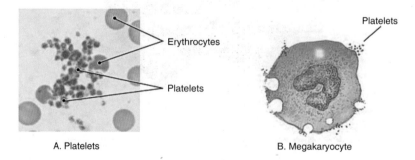

A. Platelets

B. Megakaryocyte

Figure 6-5 Platelets
A. Platelets seen in a blood smear under the microscope.
B. A megakaryocyte releases platelets.

Functions of Blood

Blood, which is a liquid connective tissue, has three general functions:

1. Transportation. As you just learned, blood transports oxygen from the lungs to the cells of the body and carbon dioxide from the body cells to the lungs for exhalation. It carries nutrients from the gastrointestinal tract to body cells and hormones from endocrine glands to other body cells. Blood also transports heat and waste products to various organs for elimination from the body.

2. Regulation. Circulating blood helps maintain **homeostasis** of all body fluids. Blood helps regulate pH through the use of **buffers**. It also helps adjust body temperature through the heat-absorbing and coolant properties of the water in blood plasma and its variable rate of flow through the skin, where excess heat can be lost from the blood to the environment. In addition, blood **osmotic** pressure influences the water content of cells, mainly through interactions of dissolved ions and proteins.

3. Protection. Blood can clot, which protects against its excessive loss from the cardiovascular system after an injury. In addition, its white blood cells protect against disease by carrying on **phagocytosis**. Several types of blood protein, including antibodies, **interferons** and **complement**, help protect against disease in a variety of ways.

The Circulatory Circuits

The cardiovascular system delivers oxygen and nutrients to the tissues and carries away waste materials to be eliminated by organs such as lungs, liver and kidneys. This system is required to function under various normalised and diseased conditions. The pulmonary and systemic circulations together help in fulfilling this role. Pulmonary circulation is a low resistance, high **capacitance** bed, and systemic circulation, in comparison, is a relatively high resistance vascular bed. The deoxygenated blood from the superior vena cava (from upper extremities, head, neck and chest wall), inferior vena cava (trunk, abdominal and pelvic organs and lower extremities) and the coronary sinus (from myocardium) reaches the right atrium (RA). The RA is filled with deoxygenated blood, increasing pressure in the atrial chamber. When the atrial pressure exceeds the pressure in the right ventricle (RV), the tricuspid valve opens allowing this blood to enter the RV. As a result of this filling, and as the RV starts to contract, the pressure in the RV builds up forcing the tricuspid valve to close and the pulmonary valve to open, thereby ejecting the blood into the pulmonary arteries and lungs. The oxygenated blood from the lungs reaches the left atrium (LA) via the pulmonary veins and as a result, pressure in LA builds up and when it exceeds that of the left ventricle (LV), the mitral valve opens, allowing the blood to enter the LV. When the blood fills the LV, and as the LV starts to contract, the LV chamber pressure increase forces the mitral valve to close and aortic valve to open, thus ejecting blood into the aorta, to be distributed throughout the body.

Checking Circulation

The alternate expansion and recoil of elastic arteries after each systole of the left ventricle creates a traveling pressure wave that is called the pulse. The pulse is strongest in the arteries closest to the heart, becomes weaker in the arterioles, and disappears altogether in the capillaries. The pulse may be felt in any artery that lies near the surface of the body that can be compressed against a bone or other firm structure.

The pulse rate normally is the same as the heart rate, about 70 to 80 beats per minute at rest. **Tachycardia** is a rapid resting heart or pulse rate over 100 beats/min. **Bradycardia** is a slow resting heart or pulse rate under 50 beats/min. Endurance-trained athletes normally exhibit bradycardia.

In clinical use, the term blood pressure usually refers to the pressure in arteries generated by the left ventricle during systole and the pressure remaining in the arteries when the ventricle is in diastole. Blood pressure is usually measured in the **brachial** artery in the left arm.

Vocabulary

agranulocyte [əˈɡrænjʊləʊˌsaɪt]   a white blood cell without granules in its cytoplasm

alkaline [ˈælkəlaɪn]   having a pH greater than 7

anucleate [eɪˈnjuːkliːɪt]   being without a nucleus

brachial [ˈbreɪkɪəl]   of or relating to an arm

bradycardia [ˌbrædɪˈkɑːdɪə]   abnormally slow heartbeat

buffer [ˈbʌfə(r)]   a solution that resists a change in acidity when an acid or base is added to it, or a substance that facilitates this resistance

capacitance [kəˈpæsɪtəns]   the property of being able to store an electric charge

complement [ˈkɒmplɪmənt]   a complex system of proteins found in blood plasma that are sequentially activated and play various roles in the immune response, including lysing bacterial cell membranes, making pathogens more susceptible to phagocyte, and recruiting inflammatory cells to sites of infection or injury

cytoplasm [ˈsaɪtəʊplæzəm]   the protoplasm of a cell contained within the cell membrane but excluding the nucleus

diapedesis [ˌdaɪəpəˈdiːsɪs]   the movement or passage of blood cells, especially white blood cells, through intact capillary walls into surrounding body tissue

elastin [ɪˈlæstɪn]   a protein similar to collagen that is the principal structural component of elastic fibers

erythrocyte [ɪˈrɪθrəsaɪt]   red blood cell

fibrin [ˈfaɪbrɪn]   an elastic, insoluble, whitish protein produced by the action of thrombin on fibrinogen and forming an interlacing fibrous network in the coagulation of blood

granulocyte [ˈɡrænjʊlə(ʊ)ˌsaɪt]   any of a group of white blood cells having granules in the cytoplasm

hematocrit [ˈhemətəʊkrɪt]   the percentage by volume of packed red blood cells in a given sample of blood after centrifugation

hemoglobin [ˌhiːməʊˈɡləʊbɪn]   the protein in the red blood cells of vertebrates that carries oxygen from the lungs to tissues and that consists of four polypeptide subunits, each of which is bound to an iron-containing heme molecule

homeostasis [ˌhəʊmɪəˈsteɪsɪs]   a state of equilibrium, as in an organism or cell, maintained by self-regulating processes

homeostatic [ˌhəʊmɪəˈsteɪtɪk]   related to or characterized by homeostasis

hormone [ˈhɔːməʊn]   a chemical substance produced in an endocrine gland and transported in the blood to a certain tissue, on which it exerts a specific effect

interferon [ˌɪntəˈfɪərɒn]   any of a family of proteins made by cells in response to virus infection that prevent the growth of the virus

leukocyte [ˈljuːkəʊsaɪt]   white blood cell

megakaryocyte [megəˈkærɪəʊsaɪt]   a large cell of the bone marrow that has a lobulated nucleus and releases platelets into the bloodstream

multinucleate [ˌmʌltɪˈnjuːklɪɪt]   having two or more nuclei

nutrient [ˈnjuːtrɪənt]   any substance that can be metabolized by an organism to give energy and build tissue

organelle [ˌɔːgəˈnel]   a structural and functional unit, such as a mitochondrion, in a cell or unicellular organism

osmotic [ɒzˈmɒtɪk]   relating to osmosis

phagocytosis [ˌfægə(ʊ)saɪˈtəʊsɪs]   the engulfing of microorganisms or other cells and foreign particles by phagocytes

plasma [ˈplæzmə]   the clear, yellowish fluid portion of blood, lymph, or intramuscular fluid in which cells are suspended

platelet [ˈpleɪtlɪt]   a minute cell occurring in the blood of vertebrates and involved in clotting of the blood

tachycardia [ˌtækɪˈkɑːdɪə]   abnormally rapid heartbeat (over 100 beats per minute)

viscosity [vɪsˈkɒsɪti]   the property of being viscous

viscous [ˈvɪskəs]   having a relatively high resistance to flow

Task 1

Directions: *Select the letter of the choice that best completes the statement or answers the question.*

(1) Blood is a complex _____ tissue in which the formed elements are suspended in plasma.

  A. connective   B. nervous   C. muscle   D. epithelial

(2) The formed elements do NOT include _____.

  A. red blood cells B. white blood cells   C. platelets   D. plasma

(3) Red blood cells are mainly responsible for transporting _____.

  A. nutrients   B. proteins   C. minerals   D. oxygen

(4) Which cells are the only complete cells in blood?

  A. Erythrocytes.   B. Leukocytes.   C. Thrombocytes.   D. Megakaryocytes.

(5) Leukocytes help defend the body against damage by _____.

  A. bacteria   B. viruses   C. parasites   D. all of the above

(6) White blood cells can be classified into _____ by staining characteristics.

A. granulocytes and agranulocytes   B. myeloid and lymphoid cells

C. polymorphonuclear and mononuclear cells   D. defense cells and phagocytes

(7) The functions of the blood include the following EXCEPT _____.

A. transportation   B. regulation   C. secretion   D. protection

(8) The deoxygenated blood from the superior vena cava, inferior vena cava and the coronary sinus reaches the _____.

A. left atrium   B. right atrium   C. left ventricle   D. right ventricle

(9) The oxygenated blood from the lungs reaches the _____ via the pulmonary veins.

A. left atrium   B. right atrium   C. left ventricle   D. right ventricle

(10) You can take your _____ using the radial artery in your wrist or the carotid artery in your neck.

A. blood sample   B. pulse   C. blood pressure   D. breath

Task 2

Directions: *Label the blood circulation.*

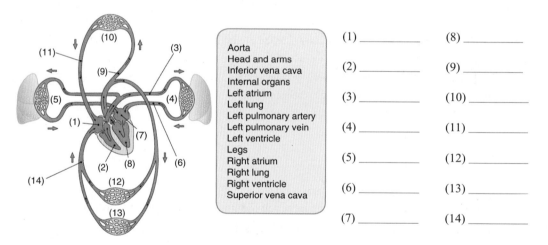

Aorta
Head and arms
Inferior vena cava
Internal organs
Left atrium
Left lung
Left pulmonary artery
Left pulmonary vein
Left ventricle
Legs
Right atrium
Right lung
Right ventricle
Superior vena cava

(1) _____   (8) _____

(2) _____   (9) _____

(3) _____   (10) _____

(4) _____   (11) _____

(5) _____   (12) _____

(6) _____   (13) _____

(7) _____   (14) _____

Task 3

Directions: *Fill in the following table based on the text above or relevant information from the Internet and then talk about the blood.*

Items	Notes
(1) composition of whole blood	
(2) composition of plasma	
(3) structure and function of erythrocytes	
(4) types and functions of leukocytes	
(5) structure and function of platelets	
(6) functions of blood	

(to be continued)

(7) pulmonary circulation	
(8) systemic circulation	
(9) pulse	
(10) blood pressure	

Task 4

Directions: *Match each of the following terms in Column A with its definition in Column B.*

A	B
(1) plasma	A. any of a group of white blood cells having granules in the cytoplasm
(2) platelet	B. a minute cell occurring in the blood of vertebrates and involved in clotting of the blood
(3) anucleate	C. having a relatively high resistance to flow
(4) hemoglobin	D. being without a nucleus
(5) granulocyte	E. abnormally rapid heartbeat
(6) homeostasis	F. the clear, yellowish fluid portion of blood, lymph, or intramuscular fluid in which cells are suspended
(7) viscous	G. a state of equilibrium, as in an organism or a cell, maintained by self-regulating processes
(8) phagocytosis	H. the engulfing of microorganisms or other cells and foreign particles by phagocytes
(9) tachycardia	I. the protein in the red blood cells of vertebrates that carries oxygen from the lungs to tissues and that consists of four polypeptide subunits, each of which is bound to an iron-containing heme molecule
(10) bradycardia	J. abnormally slow heartbeat

Medical Terminology

Roots	Terminology	Term Analysis	Definition
alkaline			
bas(o) [beɪsəʊ]	basophilia [ˌbeɪsəˈfɪliə] basophilic [beɪsəˈfɪlɪk]	phil=love, attract	
cell			
cyt(o) [saɪtəʊ]	cytology [saɪˈtɒlədʒi] cytoplasm [ˈsaɪtəʊplæzəm]		
red			
erythr(o) [ɪˈrɪθrəʊ]	erythrocyte [ɪˈrɪθrəsaɪt] erythroblast [ɪˈrɪθrə(ʊ)blæst]	blast=immature cell	

(to be continued)

granules			
granul(o) [ˈɡrænjʊləʊ]	granulocyte [ˈɡrænjʊlə(ʊ)ˌsaɪt] agranulocyte [əˈɡrænjʊləʊˌsaɪt]		
blood			
hem(o) [hi:məʊ]	hemolysis [hi:ˈmɒlɪsɪs] hemorrhage [ˈhemərɪdʒ]	-lysis=dissolving, destruction	
hemat(o) [ˈhemətəʊ]	hematocrit [ˈhemətəʊkrɪt] hematology [ˌhi:məˈtɒlədʒɪ]		
nucleus			
kary(o) [ˈkærɪəʊ]	karyotype [ˈkærɪə(ʊ)taɪp] megakaryocyte [meɡəˈkærɪəʊsaɪt]		
nucle(o) [ˈnju:klɪəʊ]	polymorphonuclear [ˌpɒlɪˌmɔ:fə(ʊ)ˈnju:klɪə] anucleate [eɪˈnju:kli:ɪt]	poly=many morph(o)=shape, form	
white			
leuk(o) [lju:kəʊ]	leukemia [lu:ˈki:mɪə] leukopenia [ˌlju:kəʊˈpi:nɪə]	-pen= deficiency	
neutral			
neutr(o) [nju:trəʊ]	neutrophil [ˈnju:trə(ʊ)fɪl] neutropenia [ˌnju:trə(ʊ)ˈpi:nɪə]		
eat/swallow			
phag(o) [fæɡəʊ]	phagocyte [ˈfæɡəsaɪt] phagocytosis [ˌfæɡə(ʊ)saɪˈtəʊsɪs]		
clot			
thromb(o) [θrɒmbəʊ]	thrombus [ˈθrɒmbəs] thrombosis [θrɒmˈbəʊsɪs]		

Vocabulary Study

Task 1

Directions: *Match each of the following terms with its definition and underline the strong part of each word where there are two or more syllables.*

(1) neutrophil	A. a large phagocytic leucocyte with a spherical nucleus and clear cytoplasm
(2) basophil	B. leukocyte with granules that are stained with basic dyes
(3) eosinophil	C. leukocyte found in lymphoid tissue and blood
(4) monocyte	D. leukocyte that stains weakly with both acidic and basic dyes
(5) lymphocyte	E. leukocyte with granules that are stained by acid dyes

(6) erythrocyte	A. a white blood cell having granules in the cytoplasm
(7) thrombocyte	B. white blood cell
(8) leukocyte	C. a white blood cell without granule in the cytoplasm
(9) granulocyte	D. platelet
(10) agranulocyte	E. red blood cell

Task 2

Directions: *Fill in the blanks with appropriate words.*

(1) A person with anemia is deficient in _____.

(2) Someone who has hemophilia suffers from excessive _____ caused by hereditary lack of blood clotting factors.

(3) The engulfing of foreign particles by a cell, such as a white blood cell, is called_____.

(4) The protein in the red blood cells of vertebrates that carries oxygen is called_____.

(5) Erythrocytes are anucleate; that is, they lack _____.

(6) A(n) _____ is a clot of coagulated blood that forms within a blood vessel or inside the heart and remains at the site of its formation, often impeding the flow of blood.

(7) An increase in the number of basophils in the circulating blood is called _____.

(8) Erythroblast is a nucleated cell occurring in bone _____ as the earliest recognizable cell of the erythrocytic series.

(9) _____ is the branch of medical science concerned with diseases of the blood and blood-forming tissues.

(10) Platelets are fragments of bizarre multinucleate cells called _____.

Task 3

Directions: Write a word for each of the following definitions using the word parts provided.

leuk(o)	hem(o)	granul(o)	erythr(o)	thromb(o)
-lytic	-emia	-poietin	-cytosis	-poiesis

(1) production of blood cells_____

(2) dissolving a blood clot_____

(3) a hormone that stimulates red blood cell production_____

(4) a neoplastic overgrowth of white blood cells_____

(5) an increase in the number of granulocytes in the blood_____

hem(o)	leuk(o)	erythr(o)	hyper-	thromb(o)	cyt(o)
-osis	-stasis	-penia	-emia	-poiesis	glyc(o)

(6) the stoppage of bleeding _____

(7) an abnormal reduction of the number of thrombocytes in the blood_____

(8) an increase in the number of leukocytes in the blood_____

(9) formation of red blood cells_____

(10) excess of glucose in the blood_____

leuk(o)	erythr(o)	thromb(o)	hypoglyc(o)	hemoglobin(o)
-cyte	-pathy	-penia	-poiesis	-emia

(11) the presence of abnormal hemoglobins in the blood_____

(12) production of platelets_____

(13) the red blood cells_____

(14) an abnormal reduction of the number of leukocytes in the blood_____

(15) low blood sugar_____

Case Study 6-1

Blood Replacement

C.L., a 16-YO girl, sustained a ruptured liver when she hit a tree while sledding. Emergency surgery was needed to stop the internal bleeding. During surgery, the ruptured segment of the liver was removed, and the laceration was sutured with a heavy, absorbable suture on a large smooth needle. Before surgery, her hemoglobin was 10.2 g/dL, but the reading decreased to 7.6 g/dL before hemostasis was attained. Cell salvage, or autotransfusion, was set up. In this procedure, the free blood was suctioned from her abdomen and mixed with an anticoagulant (heparin). The RBCs were washed in a sterile centrifuge with NS and transfused back to her through tubing fitted with a filter. She also received six units of homologous, leukocyte-reduced whole blood, five units of fresh frozen plasma, and two units of platelets. During the surgery, the CRNA repeatedly tested her Hgb and Hct as well as prothrombin time and partial thromboplastin time to monitor her clotting mechanisms.

C.L. is B-positive. Fortunately, there was enough B-positive blood in the hospital blood bank for her surgery. The lab informed her surgeon that they had two units of B-negative and six units of O-negative blood, which she could have received safely if she needed more blood during the night. However, her hemoglobin level increased to 12 g/dL, and she was stable during her recovery. She was monitored for DIC and pulmonary emboli.

Task 4

Directions: *Select the best answer to the questions or statement based on the information provided in the case of blood replacement.*

(1) Why did C.L. undertake surgery?

    A. To get a new liver.   B. To receive more blood.

    C. To replace all the blood.   D. To stop hemorrhage in the liver.

(2) The removal of the liver is called _____.

    A. hepatitis   B. hepatomegaly   C. hepatopathy   D. hepatectomy

(3) The unit for hemoglobin measurement (g/dL) stands for _____.

    A. grains per deciliter   B. grams per 100 mL

    C. grains in a decathlon   D. grams in decimal point

(4) An anticoagulant is a drug that _____.

    A. makes blood clot   B. increases blood flow

    C. interferes with blood clotting   D. helps produce more blood

(5) What does the acronym NS stand for?

    A. Nutritional solution.   B. Normal saline.

    C. Nutritional substances.   D. Normal samples.

(6) In homologous blood transfusions, a person receives _____.

    A. his own blood   B. an animal's blood

    C. blood donated by another person   D. synthetic blood

(7) For patients who lose clotting ability, effective therapy would be replacement of _____.

    A. RBCs   B. platelets   C. leukocytes   D. iron supplements

(8) The best blood for C. L. is _____.

    A. B-positive   B. B-negative   C. A-positive   D. A-negative

(9) C. L. received the following EXCEPT _____during the surgery.

    A. whole blood   B. plasma   C. platelets   D. bone marrow

(10) Which of the following is known as the universal blood type because it is safe for everyone to receive?

    A. O-negative.   B. A-negative.   C. B-negative.   D. AB-negative.

Case Study 6-2

Acute Myelocytic Leukemia

This 58-year-old man was admitted because of recurrent fever, chills, and night sweat for two weeks. Six weeks before admission, he was suspected as myelodysplastic syndrome (MDS) in a health examination and went to our outpatient clinic for consultation when he was asymptomatic except for dizziness and weakness. Complete blood count found megaloblastic anemia and bone marrow aspiration revealed abnormal localization of immature precursor. So MDS was diagnosed and he was given folic acid, vitamin B12 and prednisone, as well as interferon. Two weeks before admission, he developed chills, fever, night sweat and malodorous discharge from a spontaneous presacral ulcer, associated with mild local pain. Vancomycin, levofloxacin, and metronidazole were given intravenously. The fever resolved on the seventh day but relapsed 6 days later and the white-cell count rose to 88×10^9/L with 46% blasts. The peripheral-blood smear contained immature monocytoid cells. The specimen obtained from the bone marrow biopsy was markedly hypercellular and contained predominantly large cells with folded nuclei and moderate amounts of pale cytoplasm containing Auer rods, the characteristic of monoblasts. Dysplasia was present in all three cell lines, as shown by hypogranular neutrophils, small megakaryocytes with hypolobulated nuclei, and nuclear irregularity in the few erythroid elements identified. Immunophenotyping of the bone marrow aspiration by flow cytometry revealed $CD45^+$, dimly $CD34^+$, HLA-DR$^+$, blasts expressing the myeloid markers CD33, myeloperoxidase, CD117 and the monocytic markers CD64 and CD14. Cytogenetic analysis revealed a normal karyotype (46, XY). The peripheral-blood smear and the bone marrow aspiration and biopsy specimen suggested acute myelocytic leukemia (AML).

Task 5

Directions: Write a word or phrase from the case study that means the same as each of the following.

(1) pertaining to a young cell of the granulocytic series, occurring normally in bone marrow

(2) related to an abnormality of development of myelocytes and other cells in the bone marrow

(3) pertaining to an abnormally large immature red blood cell

(4) having a bad smell

(5) before the sacrum

(6) resembling a large white blood cell that circulates in the blood and then migrates into the tissues, where it matures into a macrophage

(7) with less granules

(8) with less lobes

(9) the counting of blood cells

(10) the number and shape of chromosomes in the nucleus of a cell

Medical Term Extension

Basic Surgical Instrument

A surgery cannot be carried out without medical tests and tools. There are a variety of surgical instruments, each designed for a specific purpose. Some are used for making an incision while others are made to hold tissues. Using them correctly is necessary to prevent any irreversible damage to the internal organs of the body.

Basic Surgical Instruments and Their Uses

Information about the most frequently used surgical instruments is given below:

Scalpel

This is a surgical knife that comes with a sharp stainless steel blade. Whether it is a minor or a major surgery, a correct surgical incision is a must, which is not possible without a scalpel. Each and every surgery has its own specific needs. For instance, a minor surgery will require a small incision whereas a major surgery may demand an incision deep into the skin tissues. So taking this into consideration, scalpels are manufactured in a variety of sizes. The blades of scalpel are detachable and many times this instrument is designed for one time use only.

Surgical Staples

Talking about list of surgical instruments and one simply cannot forget to mention about surgical staples. Normally, an incision made or an open wound that occurs during surgery cannot be left open as it can trigger internal bleeding. A common practice is to seal these cuts using stitches but nowadays surgeons prefer to use surgical staples instead of stitches. The main advantage is that the possibility of blood leaking from a wound closed by a surgical staple is minimal. Apart from closing the incision, surgical staples are also useful to reattach and remove portions of certain organs. For instance, a bowel surgery may demand cutting certain parts of the intestine and reconnecting the remaining portion of the intestine. This can be effectively and precisely done using surgical staples.

Surgical Suture

As we all know, during surgery incisions are made to carry out the procedure. Surgical sutures, which are nothing but stitches, are commonly used to reconnect the tissues so as to close the incision after the surgical procedure is over. Sutures also help to join wound edges after an injury. This closing of wound helps to facilitate healing of the injury. Modern sutures are made from synthetic material that can be either absorbable or non-absorbable one.

Absorbable Sutures

Absorbable sutures are absorbed by the body over a course of time. The duration of absorption varies according to the type of suture material but lasts anywhere between 10 days to 2 months. When the suture is placed deep inside the body or the patient is not in a position to visit the hospital again to remove sutures, then the absorbable sutures are used. Absorbable sutures are primarily constructed from synthetic material like polylactic acid, polyglycolic acid, and caprolactone.

Non-absorbable Sutures

Non-absorbable sutures are non-biodegradable; hence cannot be broken down by the body and absorbed. The material used in making non-absorbable sutures is usually polypropylene, nylon, or polyester. Stainless steel wires that exhibit high tensile strength are often preferred to close the sternum following heart surgery. In general, non-absorbable sutures have an advantage over their counterparts, as they cause minimal scarring. Usually these sutures are removed after a specified duration but in some cases, they are allowed to remain in the position.

Hemostat

During any surgical procedure, some amount of bleeding is there for sure. A slight incision here and there is followed by bleeding. In order to prevent any sort of major complications, the surgeon often uses a hemostat. This is a clamp-like surgical tool that is utilized to constrict a blood vessel, which helps to minimize or stop the flow of blood during any surgical procedure.

Dilator

Surgical procedures involving the esophagus, urethra, or the cervix often require the surgeon to enlarge the opening of these tubular structures. This can be done using dilators, instruments that expand the passage, thereby allowing the surgeon to access the organ and perform the surgeon properly. These tools induce dilation to open up a tube, duct or cavity for surgical purposes.

Scissors

This surgical instrument is mainly used to cut body tissues. Scissors used in surgery come in two main types: Mayo and Metzenbaum scissors. When it comes to cutting or dissecting soft delicate tissues, surgeons prefer the Metzenbaum scissors. The Mayo scissors are used for cutting hard tissues such as joints. Thick tissues located in the breast and the muscles can also be cut using Mayo scissors. Usually, these scissors are made up of stainless steel and are manufactured in variable lengths.

Needle Holder

As we all know, stitching the body tissues that are cut at the time of surgery is a very important task. Even a slight mistake while sewing the tissue is likely to make the patient uncomfortable days after completing the surgery. An improperly sewn skin tissue can be a cause of great pain and may require another surgery to correct it. To avoid all these complications and to carry out sewing of tissues accurately, surgeons often make use of needle holders. These instruments allow the surgeon to hold the needle firmly while stitching the required tissue.

A needle holder that has a shape similar to a scissor, consists of straight, smooth jaws, joints and handles. It comes with a tungsten carbide inserts that are attached at the end of both the jaws. They ensure that the needle does not move while sewing tissues. In simple words, these instruments are designed to provide a strong grip on the needle, thereby substantially reducing the chances of any error during this stage of surgery.

Forceps

Forceps are like kitchen tongs that allow the surgeon to grasp and hold the skin tissues firmly. Whether it is holding a part of intestine or clamping the arteries during operation, one can always rely on these forceps. This surgical instrument comes in a range of sizes so that the surgeon can choose one depending upon his specific needs. Forceps that are designed to hold a baby's head are quite large and their main purpose is to safely remove the baby from the birth canal during a cesarean.

Curette

This surgical tool resembling to a spoon is used for taking out unwanted tissue from internal body cavities. Using the tool, the surgeon simply scrapes to scoop out the abnormal tissue. Cleaning procedure such as removing cancer growth may require use of curette.

Retractors

When an incision is made, it has to be kept open during surgery. This job of keeping the incision wide open is done by retractors. These instruments are used to pull back the tissues so that the surgeon can easily access the operation site and perform the surgery without any hindrance. Sometimes even the organs have to be held back using retractors, so as to expose the surgical site to the desired level. Retractors are made available in different sizes and shapes. Also, there are different types of retractors and each one is designed to retract a specific organ. For instance, lung retractors may be used to push aside the lungs gently for getting an unobstructed view of the surgical site. So, be it a gallbladder surgery or a breast reduction surgery, it cannot be done without retractors.

Surgical Elevator

When it comes to performing oral surgery such as tooth extraction, it is not possible without a surgical elevator. This tool is commonly used in dentistry for removing or separating affected teeth from their sockets. It is also used for separating bones from their tissues.

Probe

A probe is a long, flexible surgical tool that has a blunt end and is used for probing a wound and body cavities such as a sinus tract. The instrument helps to evaluate the wound such as how deep the wound is. The direction of wound can also be assessed using this tool. As the instrument is inserted in the wound or cavity, excessive usage can trigger pain and cause pain in patients.

These are some of the basic surgical instruments and their uses. Keep in mind that it is important to choose a surgical tool that is appropriate for the procedure. Choosing the wrong tools can not only be traumatic for the patient but can also prevent the surgeon from doing his best work.

Task 6

Directions: *Name the following items in English.*

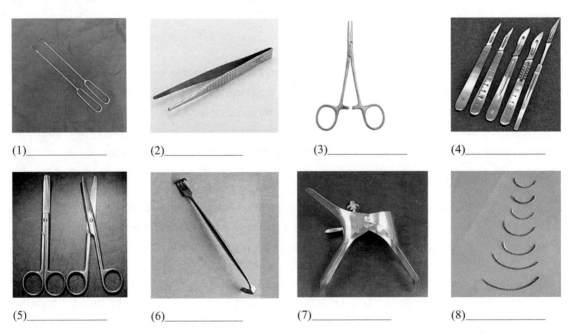

(1)_____ (2)_____ (3)_____ (4)_____

(5)_____ (6)_____ (7)_____ (8)_____

Writing

Tips for Writing the Perfect IMRaD Manuscript

To ensure that your manuscript conveys your ideas effectively, it is essential for you to structure it well. Many journals expect scientific research papers to be written in the traditional format, which is also referred to as the IMRaD format (Introduction, Materials and Methods, Results, and Discussion). Here, I will cover some quick tips on writing each of the IMRaD sections to help you ensure that your manuscript communicates your research effectively.

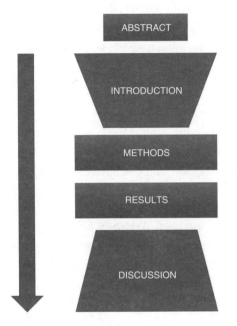

Different journals have variations on the model. For example, sometimes the Results and Discussion sections are combined. However, the general order above is a good guide to follow.

From the diagram, you will see that the Introduction and Discussion have funnel shapes which are mirror images of each other. This is because the Introduction goes from the general to the specific areas which will be covered in the article. The Discussion then goes from the specific findings to the broader implications of these findings. The Discussion often incorporates the Conclusion.

Introduction

The Introduction of your research paper should clearly explain what you are studying and why. It is important for you to set context for your study, too. Your readers need to understand what you are trying to say. Use general language in this section and develop your ideas logically to build the story behind your study.

Writing the Introduction: The Introduction answers the question W-H-Y.

Begin by describing the problem that you wanted to solve through the piece of research you are writing about. Explain why that problem is important. As Peter Medawar warns in his *Advice to a Young Scientist*, "the problem must be such that it matters what the answer is — whether to science generally or to mankind." Next, briefly review what has been done so far to solve the problem. Finally, introduce the study by pointing out what is different about it compared to past research.

Materials and Methods

The Methods section should include what you did and how you went about conducting your research. A research that is well conducted should be replicable. Any other researcher should be able to reproduce the results you achieved by following the methods you have detailed in your manuscript.

> **Writing the Materials and Methods section: The section on Materials and Methods answers the question H-O-W.**
>
> Include enough detail so that others can repeat the experiment if they wish to do so. Give sources of material, make and model of equipment, quantities, duration, reason, etc. All research is expected to be reproducible, which is why this section is particularly important. Describe what the "treatments" were and how you arranged for appropriate "controls" so that valid comparisons can be made between these two sets. Also, this is perhaps the easiest section to write, and it is a good idea to start your writing with this section.

Results

The Results section indicates whether you were able to solve the problem you outlined in the Introduction. It is essential to include complete details along with data in this section. Highlighting the most significant findings or organizing them into sections will ensure that you have covered all the relevant information.

> **Writing the Results section: The Results section answers the question W-H-A-T.**
>
> State only the results; leave comments and explanations for the Discussion section. Use tables and charts as appropriate, but do not duplicate the data by presenting the same data once as a table and once as a graph or by repeating the graphical data in the text. In theory, this section can be the shortest of the IMRaD sections because a lot of the information can be presented in tables and/or figures.

Discussion

The Discussion section is also closely tied to the Introduction. Research does not end with conducting a study and extracting results. The implications and meaning of your findings also need to be discussed in order to understand the impact your research has had.

The Conclusion should state the primary conclusions of your study with regard to the problem you started out with. In short, write what you learned through your study here. In the case of some research fields or topics of study, it is essential to include an explanation of how and why you arrived at the present conclusion.

> **Writing the Discussion section: The Discussion section answers the most important question, namely, S-O W-H A-T.**
>
> Explain what the results mean and how they are important. Compare the results with earlier findings; explain contradictory results, if any. If some results did not attain statistical significance, explain that any differences seen may have been due to chance. Outline the limitations of your study, and suggest a future line of work. Finally, sum up with a conclusion.

To ensure that your reader (including the journal editor and reviewer) is able to understand the full implications of your work, ensure that your manuscript is well-structured and that each of the IMRaD elements is clearly written and organized.

Task 1

Directions: *Discuss whether the following are DOs or DON'Ts.*

Introduction	☐ Describe the rationale for undertaking the study.
	☐ Explain how the research makes an important contribution to the field or advances knowledge.
	☐ State the research question clearly.
	☐ Explain the theoretical framework that the study is based on.
	☐ Provide a background of the problem or issue that your research aims to understand or resolve, citing studies to support your arguments.
	☐ Summarize the current state of knowledge on the topic, citing studies as appropriate.
	☐ Review all studies that have ever been published on the topic.
Materials and Methods	☐ Provide full details of all methods, techniques, and instruments.
	☐ Include photograph or diagram of the experimental setup.
	☐ Describe the questionnaire, survey, or other data collection instruments.
	☐ Provide or cite studies that support the validity and reliability of the analysis methods and instruments.
	☐ Describe the lab settings or environment.
	☐ Explain the analysis methods and why you chose them.
	☐ Exclude important details simply to avoid a lengthy description of the methods.
Results	☐ Use tables and figures effectively to present results in a manner that's easy to understand at a glance.
	☐ Describe the actual data rather than provide generalizations.
	☐ State the main findings in the text.
	☐ Highlight any unexpected or surprising results in the text.
	☐ Explain what the results are saying, rather them simply stating the statistical data (e.g., "X was found to substantially increase with Y [followed by statistical data]" rather than "X and Y had a positive correlation of .73").
	☐ If you have illustrated the results of your study in figures and tables, include detailed descriptions of these results in the text.

(to be continued)

Discussion	☐ Start by stating whether your hypothesis was supported.
	☐ Interpret the results: what do the results imply?
	☐ Relate your findings to those of previous studies, for example, whether your results support or deviate from results in previous studies.
	☐ Explain how the study adds to previous knowledge.
	☐ Remember to mention any possible alternative explanations for the results.
	☐ Address the limitations of the study.
	☐ Simply repeat the results again.
	☐ Draw conclusions that are not supported by the data.
Conclusion	☐ Explain what you've learned from the study.
	☐ Ensure that the conclusion is directly related to your research question and stated purpose of the study.
	☐ Elaborate on the broader implications of the research.
	☐ Suggest specific future avenues of research to advance the knowledge you've gained from the study or answer questions that your study did not address.
	☐ Oversell your research or "overgeneralize" the results, that is, stretch the study findings to provide suggestions or conclusions that the research doesn't really support.
	☐ Simply summarize the results.

Task 2

Directions: Read the section of Introduction and think about the funneling writing process.

(A) Apolipoprotein (apo) E is a 34-kD protein component of lipoproteins that mediates their binding to the low density lipoprotein(LDL) receptor and to LDL receptor-related protein(LRP)[1-4]. (B) Apolipoprotein E is a major apolipoprotein in the central nervous system, where it is thought to redistribute lipoprotein cholesterol among the neurons and their supporting cells, thus maintaining cholesterol homeostasis[5-7]. (C) In addition to this function, apo E in the peripheral nervous system redistributes lipids during regeneration[8-10].

(D) There are three common isoforms of apo E(apoE2, apoE3, and apoE4) that are the products of three alleles (ε2, ε3, and ε4) at a single gene locus on chromosome 19[11]. (E) Apo E3, the most common isoform, has cysteine and arginine at positions 112 and 158, respectively[1, 12]. (F)ApoE2 has cysteine at both of these positions[1, 12]. (G)ApoE4 has arginine at both[1, 12].

(H)The apoE4 allele (ε4) is a major risk factor for sporadic and familial late-onset Alzheimer's disease[13—16]. (I)In support of this finding, apoE4 immunoreactivity has been detected in both the amyloid plaques and the intracellular neurofibrillary tangles seen in postmortem examinations of brains from Alzheimer's disease patients[17, 18].

(J) The mechanism by which apoE4 might contribute to Alzheimer's disease is unknown.

(K) However, our recent data demonstrating that apoE4 stunts the outgrowth of neuritis from neurons of the dorsal root ganglion (DRG)[19, 20] suggest that apoE4 might contribute to Alzheimer's disease by stunting the outgrowth of these neurites. (L)Our data further suggest that outgrowth might be stunted by remodeling of the cytoskeleton, specifically the microtubule system. (M)Therefore, as a step toward determining the mechanism of apoE4's contribution to Alzheimer's disease, we asked whether apoE4 inhibits outgrowth of neurites from Neuro-2a cells, a mouse neuroblastoma cell line, by remodeling the microtubule system of these cells.

Task 3

Directions: *The section of Materials and Methods may contain various types of subheadings. Read the subheadings below and determine whether they are organized in chronological order or by the type of procedure.*

Materials
Animals
Preparation
Study design
Interventions
Methods of measurement
Calculation
Analysis of Data

Trypanosomes
Stable transformation
    DNA constructs
    Transfection
T. Brucei relapse experiments
    In vivo relapse
    In vitro relapse
DNA, RNA, and protein analysis
…

Task 4

Directions: *The section of Results illustrates tables and graphs. Complete the following illustration based on tables or graphs provided.*

Table 1 Incidence of ulcer perforation 1967—1982

		>65	65—74	>75
No. of prescriptions per 1000 (Women)	1967	500		
	1982	1500		
Perforations (Women)	1967		7	10
	1982		14	33
No. of prescriptions (Men)	1967	290		
	1982	820		
Perforations (Men)	1967		36	32
	1982		28	65

Table 1 _____ trends in the frequency of hospital admission for perforated peptic ulcer in the United Kingdom _____ with changes in the annual prescription rates for non-steroidal anti-inflammatory drugs. For women over 65 the annual number of prescriptions increased from 1967 to1982, during which rates of perforation of duodenal ulcers _____ for those aged 65 to 74 and more than _____ for those aged 75 and over. For men over 65, prescriptions showed a similar increase. Although perforation rates were actually lower for those aged 65 to 74 in 1982, there was a _____ increase in those aged 75 and above.

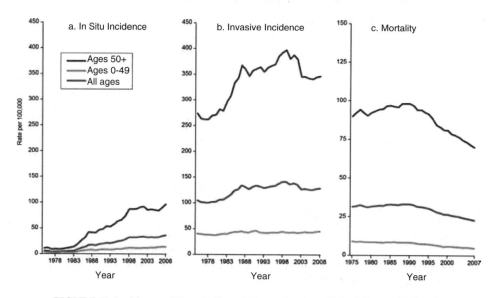

FIGURE X. Incidence of Female Breast Cancer by Age, United States, 1975 to 2008

Delay-adjusted incidence rates for in situ and invasive female breast cancer for women under age 50 years and those aged 50 years and older are _____ (presented/represented) in Figure X. In the early 1980s incidence rates of invasive breast cancer _____ (increased/fell) among both women 50 years of age and older and those aged younger than 50 years. Among women 50 years of age and older, incidence rates _____ (stabilized/reached a peak) from 1987 through 1993 and then increased again from 1993 to 1999, but at a _____ (faster/slower) rate. Between 2002 and 2003, breast cancer rates _____ (rose/dropped) _____ (sharply/gradually). Incidence rates have been stable among women aged older than 50 years since 2004. Among women aged younger than 50 years, incidence rates have _____ (fell/remained) stable since 1985. Incidence rates of in situ breast cancer rose _____ (rapidly/steadily) in the 1980s and 1990s. Since 1999, incidence rates of in situ breast cancer have stabilized in women aged 50 years and older, but _____ (continue/decline) to increase in younger women.

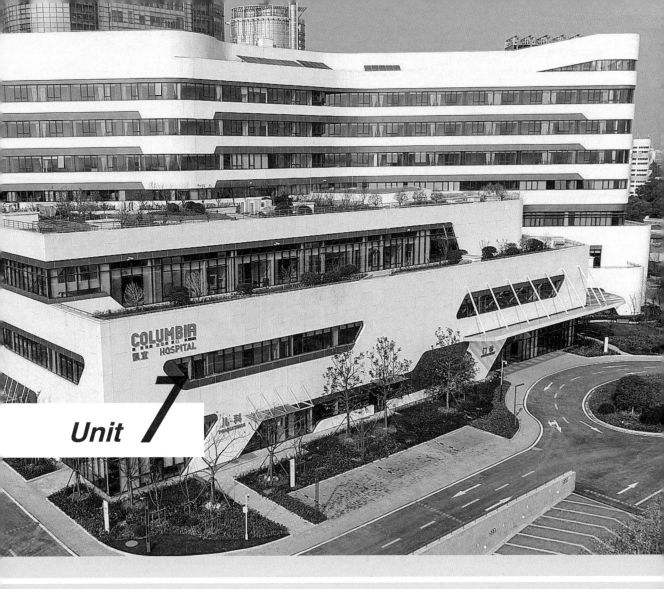

The Urinary System

√ 听力音频
√ 听力文本
√ 课件资源

Warm-up

1. What are the symptoms of some urinary diseases?

2. What can you do to prevent them?

SYMPTOMS

· Strong and frequent urge to urinate
· Bloody or dark urine with strong smell
· Burning sensation while urinating
· Pain in lower back or below the ribs
· Pain in your bladder region
· Muscle aches and abdominal pains

· Vomiting
· Chills
· High fever (over 101°F)
· Fatigue

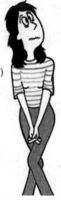

PREVENTION

· Drink eight to ten glasses of water a day
· Don't control, urinate as soon as you feel the need
· Take showers instead of baths
· Females should wipe from front to back after urinating
· Avoid the use of douches or feminine hygiene sprays

· Loose fitting clothes to promote air circulating

Theme Reading

The urinary system consists of two kidneys, two **ureters**, the **urinary bladder**, and the **urethra**. A large volume of blood flows through the kidneys, which removes substances from the blood to form urine. The urine produced by the kidneys flows through the ureters to the urinary bladder, where it is stored until it is eliminated through the urethra.

The Urinary System

Objectives

☆ *Identify the components of the urinary system.*
☆ *List the major functions of the urinary system.*
☆ *Describe the location and anatomical structure of the kidneys.*
☆ *Describe the process of urine formation in the body.*
☆ *Describe the process of urination.*

The excretory organs of the human body include the kidneys, skin, intestines and lungs. The urinary system performs the main part of the excretory function in the body. The most important excretory organs are the kidneys. If the kidneys fail to function properly, toxic wastes start to accumulate in the body.

Functions of the Urinary System

The major functions of the urinary system are performed by the kidneys, and the kidneys play the following essential roles in controlling the composition and volume of body fluids:

1. *Excretion*. The kidneys are the major excretory organs of the body. They remove waste products, many of which are toxic, from the blood. Most waste products are metabolic by-products of cells and substances absorbed from the intestine. The skin, liver, lungs and intestines eliminate some of these waste products, but they cannot compensate if the kidneys fail to function.

2. *Regulation of blood volume and pressure*. The kidneys play a major role in controlling the extracellular fluid volume in the body by producing either a large volume of **dilute** urine or a small volume of concentrated urine. Consequently, blood volume and blood pressure are regulated by the kidneys.

3. *Regulation of the concentration of solutes in the blood*. The kidneys help regulate the concentration of the major molecules and ions such as glucose, Na^+, Cl^-, K^+, Ca^{2+}, HCO_3^-, and HPO_4^{2-}.

4. *Regulation of extracellular fluid pH*. The kidneys secrete variable amounts of H^+ to help regulate extracellular fluid pH.

5. *Regulation of red blood cell synthesis*. The kidneys secrete a hormone, **erythropoietin**, which regulates the synthesis of red blood cells in bone marrow.

6. *Vitamin D synthesis*. The kidneys play an important role in controlling blood levels of Ca^{2+} by regulating the synthesis of vitamin D.

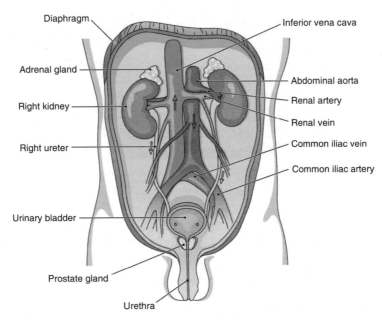

Figure 7-1 The male urinary system

Kidneys

The kidneys are bean-shaped organs resting high against the dorsal wall of the abdominal cavity; they lie on either side of the vertebral column between the **peritoneum** and the back muscles. Because the kidneys are located behind the peritoneum, they are said to be **retroperitoneal**. They are positioned between the twelfth thoracic and the third lumbar vertebrae. The right kidney is situated slightly lower than the left due to the large area occupied by the liver.

Each kidney with its blood vessels is enclosed within a mass of fat tissue called the **adipose capsule**. In turn, each kidney and adipose capsule is covered by a tough, fibrous tissue called the renal fascia.

There is an **indentation** along the **concave** medial border of the kidney called the **hilum**. The hilum is a passageway for the lymph vessel, nerves, renal artery and vein, and the ureter. At the hilum the fibrous capsule continues downward, forming the outer layer of the ureter. Cutting the kidney in half lengthwise reveals its internal structure. The upper end of each ureter flares into a **funnel**-shaped structure known as the **renal pelvis**.

The kidneys have the potential to work harder than they actually do. Under ordinary circumstances, only a portion of the **nephron** is used. Should one kidney not function, or have to be removed, more nephrons and tubules open up in the second kidney to assume the work of the nonfunctioning or missing kidney.

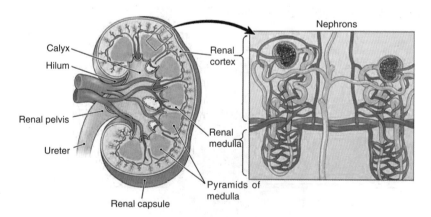

Figure 7-2 The kidney

Nephron

The nephron is the basic structural and functional unit of the kidney. Most of the nephron is located within the cortex, with only a small, tubular portion in the **medulla**. Each kidney has over one million nephrons which altogether comprise 140 miles of filters and tubes.

A nephron begins with the **afferent arteriole**, which carries blood from the renal artery. The afferent arteriole enters a double-walled hollow capsule, the **Bowman's capsule**.

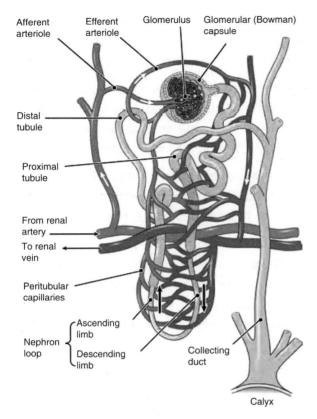

Figure 7-3 A nephron and its blood supply

Within the capsule the afferent arteriole finely divides, forming a knotty ball called the **glomerulus**, which contains some 50 separate capillaries. The combination of the Bowman's capsule and the glomerulus is known as the **renal corpuscle**. The Bowman's capsule sends off a highly convoluted tubular branch referred to as the **proximal convoluted tubule**.

The proximal convoluted tubule descends into the medulla to form the **loop of Henle**. The loop of Henle has a straight descending limb, a loop, and a straight ascending limb. When the ascending limb of Henle's loop returns to the cortex, it turns into the **distal convoluted tubule**. Eventually this convoluted tubule opens into a larger, straight vessel known as the collecting tubule. Several distal convoluted tubules join to form this single straight collection tubule. The **collecting tubule** empties into the renal pelvis, then into the ureter.

The walls of the renal tubules are surrounded by capillaries. After the afferent arteriole branches out to form the glomerulus, it leaves the Bowman's capsule as the **efferent arteriole**. The efferent arteriole branches to form the **peritubular capillaries** surrounding the renal tubules. All of these capillaries eventually join together to form a small branch of the renal vein which carries blood from the kidney.

Urine Formation in the Nephron

Each kidney has about a million nephrons, where urine formation takes place. At any given time, about 20 percent of the blood is going through the kidneys to be filtered so that the body can eliminate waste and maintain hydration, blood pH and proper levels of blood substances.

The first part of urine formation occurs in the glomeruli, which are small clumps of blood vessels. The glomeruli act as filters, allowing water, glucose, salt and waste materials to pass through to the Bowman's capsule, which surrounds each glomerulus, but preventing the red blood cells from passing. The fluid in the Bowman's capsule is referred to as the nephric **filtrate** and resembles blood plasma. It also includes **urea** produced from the **ammonia** which accumulates when the liver processes amino acids and is filtered out by the glomeruli.

About 43 gallons of fluid goes through the filtration process, but most is subsequently reabsorbed rather than being eliminated. Reabsorption occurs in the proximal tubules of the nephron, which is the portion beyond the capsule, in the loop of Henle, and in the distal and collecting tubules, which are further along the nephron beyond the loop of Henle.

Water, glucose, amino acids, sodium and other nutrients are reabsorbed into the bloodstream in the capillaries surrounding the tubules. Water moves via the process of **osmosis**: movement of water from an area of higher concentration to one of lower concentration.

Usually all the glucose is reabsorbed, but in diabetic individuals, excess glucose remains in the filtrate. Sodium and other **ions** are reabsorbed incompletely, with a greater proportion remaining in the filtrate when more is consumed in the diet, resulting in higher blood concentrations. Hormones regulate the process of active transport by which ions like sodium and **phosphorus** are reabsorbed.

Secretion is the final step in the process of urine formation. Some substances move directly from the blood in capillaries around the distal and collecting tubules into those tubules. Secretion of hydrogen ions via this process is part of the body's mechanism for maintaining proper pH, or acid-base balance. More ions are secreted when the blood is acidic, less when it is **alkaline**.

Potassium ions, calcium ions and ammonia also are secreted at this stage, as are some medications. The kidney is considered a **homeostatic** organ, one that helps maintain the chemical composition of the blood within strict limits. It does this partly by stepping up secretion of substances such as potassium and calcium when concentrations are high and by increasing reabsorption and reducing secretion when levels are low.

The urine created by this process then passes to the central part of the kidney called the pelvis, where it flows into the ureters and then the **bladder**.

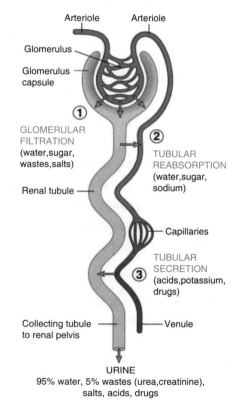

Figure 7-4 Three steps in the formation of urine

Ureters

The ureters are narrow tubes that carry urine from the kidneys to the bladder. Muscles in the ureter walls continually tighten and relax forcing urine downward, away from the kidneys. If urine backs up, or is allowed to stand still, a kidney infection can develop. About every 10 to 15 seconds, small amounts of urine are emptied into the bladder from the ureters.

Urinary Bladder

The bladder is a triangle-shaped, hollow organ located in the lower abdomen. It is held in place by **ligaments** that are attached to other organs and the pelvic bones. The bladder's walls relax and expand to store urine, and contract and flatten to empty urine through the urethra. The typical healthy adult bladder can store up to two cups of urine for two to five hours.

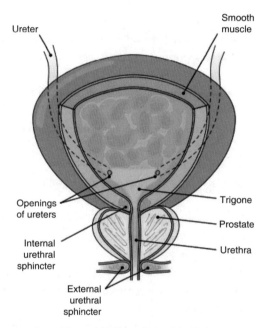

Figure 7-5 The urinary bladder

Sphincter Muscles

The sphincter muscles refer to the circular muscles that help keep urine from leaking by closing tightly like a rubber band around the opening of the bladder.

Urethra

The urethra is the tube that allows urine to pass outside the body. The brain signals the bladder muscles to tighten, which squeezes urine out of the bladder. At the same time, the brain signals the sphincter muscles to relax to let urine exit the bladder through the urethra. When all the signals occur in the correct order, normal urination occurs.

Vocabulary

adipose capsule [ˈædɪpəʊz] perirenal fat

afferent arteriole [ˈæfərənt] a blood vessel in the kidney that supplies blood to glomeruli

alkaline [ˈælkəlaɪn] having the qualities of an alkali, having a pH greater than 7.0

ammonia [əˈməʊnɪə] colorless gas or liquid that has a strong smell and taste and that is used especially in cleaning products

bladder [ˈblædə] the organ in the body that holds urine after it passes through the kidneys and before it leaves the body

Bowman's capsule [ˈkæpsjuːl] the globular dilatation forming the beginning of a renal tubule and surrounding the glomerulus, called also glomerular capsule

collecting tubule [ˈtjuːbjuːl] one of the small ducts that receive urine from several renal tubules, which join together to provide a passage for the urine to larger straight collecting tubules that open into the pelvis of the kidney

concave [ˈkɒnkeɪv] hollowed or rounded inward like the inside of a bowl

dilute [daɪˈljuːt] to make a mixture or solution less concentrated by adding a fluid

distal convoluted tubule [ˈdɪstl] a portion of kidney nephron between the loop of Henle and the collecting tubule

efferent arteriole [aːˈtɪəriəʊl] blood vessels that are part of the urinary tract, carry blood away from the glomerulus that has already been filtered

erythropoietin [ɪˌrɪθrəˈpɔɪetɪn] a hormonal substance that is formed especially in the kidney and stimulates red blood cell formation

filtrate [ˈfɪltreɪt] fluid that has passed through a filter

funnel [ˈfʌnl] a tube or pipe that is wide at the top and narrow at the bottom, used for guiding liquid or powder into a small opening

glomerulus [glɒˈmerjʊləs] a tuft of capillaries at the point of origin of each vertebrate nephron that passes a protein-free filtrate to the surrounding Bowman's capsule

hilum [ˈhaɪləm] the indented part of a kidney

homeostatic [ˌhəʊmɪəˈsteɪtɪk] maintaining relatively stable internal physiological conditions (as body temperature or the pH of blood) in higher animals under fluctuating environmental conditions

indentation [ˌɪndenˈteɪʃn] a concave cut into a surface or edge

ion [ˈaɪən] an atom or group of atoms that carries a positive or negative electric charge as a result of having lost or gained one or more electrons

ligament [ˈlɪgəmənt] the fibrous connective tissue that connects bones to other bones

loop of Henle [luːp] a U-shaped segment of the nephron in a vertebrate kidney that functions in water resorption

medulla [meˈdʌlə] the inner or deep part of an organ or structure

nephron [ˈnefrɒn] the microscopic structural and functional unit of the kidney

osmosis [ɒzˈməʊsɪs] the process that causes a liquid (especially water) to pass through the wall of a living cell

peritoneum [ˌperɪtəˈnɪəm] the smooth transparent serous membrane that lines the cavity of the abdomen of a mammal

peritubular capillary [kəˈpɪləri] any of a network of capillaries surrounding the renal tubules

phosphorus [ˈfɒsfərəs] a poisonous chemical element that glows in the dark and burns when it is touched by air

proximal convoluted tubule [ˈprɒksɪməl]   the convoluted portion of the vertebrate nephron lying between Bowman's capsule and the loop of Henle; functions in the resorption of sugar, sodium and chloride ions, and water.

renal corpuscle [ˈkɔːpʌsl]   the blood-filtering component of the nephron of the kidney

renal fascia [ˈfæʃɪə]   a layer of connective tissue encapsulating the kidneys and the adrenal glands

renal pelvis [ˈpelvɪs]   a funnel-shaped structure in each kidney that receives urine from the collecting duct for passage into the ureter

retroperitoneal [ˌretrəˌperɪtəˈnɪəl]   situated or occurring behind the peritoneum

solute [ˈsɒljuːt]   a dissolved substance

urea [jʊəˈriːə]   a water-soluble compound, that is the major nitrogenous end product of protein metabolism and is the chief nitrogenous component of the urine in mammals and certain other animals

ureter [jʊəˈriːtə]   the long, narrow duct that conveys urine from the kidney to the urinary bladder

urethra [jʊəˈriːθrə]   the canal that in most mammals carries off the urine from the bladder and in the male serves also as a passageway for semen

urinary [ˈjʊərɪnəri]   relating to, occurring in, affecting, or constituting the organs concerned with the formation and discharge of urine

Task 1

Directions: *Select the letter of the choice that best completes the statement or answers the question.*

(1) The urinary system performs the main part of the _____ in the body.
   A. filtration function   B. excretory function
   C. reproductive function   D. digestive function

(2) The excretory organs of the human body include the kidneys, skin, _____ and lungs.
   A. intestines   B. stomach   C. urinary bladder   D. gallbladder

(3) The expanded upper end of the ureter that receives urine from the kidney is called the_____.
   A. renal pelvis   B. renal fascia   C. renal corpuscle   D. renal medulla

(4) A microscopic functional unit of the kidney is the_____, which filters the blood and balances the composition of urine.
   A. calyx   B. nephron   C. tubule   D. capsule

(5) Which of the following is NOT included in the loop of Henle?
   A. A loop.   B. A descending limb.
   C. A convoluted tubule.   D. An ascending limb.

(6) The cluster of capillaries within the glomerular capsule is the_____, which passes a protein-free filtrate to the surrounding Bowman's capsule.
   A. Bowman's capsule   B. glomerulus
   C. renal corpuscle   D. loop of Henle

(7) The combination of the Bowman's capsule and the glomerulus is known as the _____.

    A. Bowman's capsule   B. glomerulus

    C. renal corpuscle   D. loop of Henle

(8) The first part of urine formation occurs in the _____.

    A. glomeruli   B. renal tubules   C. loop of Henle   D. renal pelvis

(9) _____ is the main nitrogenous waste product in the urine.

    A. Glucose   B. Urea   C. Sodium   D. Amino acid

(10) The tube that carries urine from the bladder to the outside of the body is called the_____.

    A. proximal convoluted tubule   B. collecting tubule

    C. urethra   D. ureter

Task 2

Directions: *Label the organs of the urinary system. Write the name of each numbered part on the corresponding line.*

abdominal aorta	common iliac artery	inferior vena cava
renal artery	right kidney	urethra
adrenal gland	common iliac vein	prostate gland
renal vein	right ureter	urinary bladder

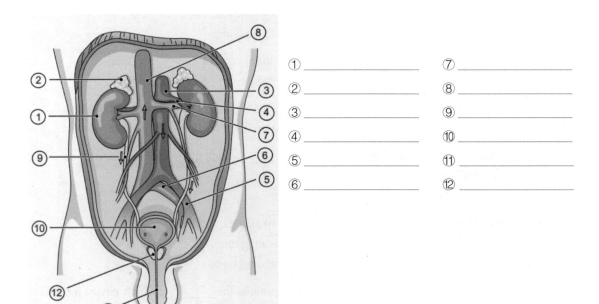

①_____   ⑦_____

②_____   ⑧_____

③_____   ⑨_____

④_____   ⑩_____

⑤_____   ⑪_____

⑥_____   ⑫_____

Task 3

Directions: *Read the following statements, and then decide whether they are true (T) or false (F).*

(1) The kidneys are the most important excretory organs of the body.

(2) The hilum is the point where blood vessels and ducts connect with the kidney.

(3) Each kidney contains more than 1 billion nephrons.

(4) The nephron, the tiny working unit of the kidney, regulates the proportion of water, waste, and other materials in urine according to the body's constantly changing needs.

(5) A nephron consists of a renal corpuscle and a renal tubule.

(6) The kidneys remove waste products from the intestine.

(7) Blood filtration occurs through the glomerulus in the nephron loop.

(8) Substances that enter the nephron can be returned to the blood through the peritubular capillaries that surround the nephron.

Task 4

Directions: *Match each of the following terms in Column A with its definition in Column B.*

A	B
(1) arteriole	A. inner region of an organ
(2) glomerulus	B. hormone secreted by the kidney that stimulates formation of red blood cells
(3) hilum	C. nitrogenous waste
(4) medulla	D. small artery
(5) calyx	E. the pale yellow slightly acid fluid excreted by the kidneys, containing waste products removed from the blood
(6) erythropoietin	F. tiny ball of capillaries in the kidney
(7) cortex	G. cup-like collecting region of the renal pelvis
(8) urine	H. depression in an organ where blood vessels and nerves enter and leave
(9) meatus	I. outer region of an organ
(10) urea	J. opening or canal

Medical Terminology

Roots	Terminology	Term Analysis	Definition
urine			
ur(o) [ˈjʊərəʊ]	uremia [jʊəˈriːmɪə] urology [jʊəˈrɒlədʒi]		
ureter			
ureter(o) [jʊəˈriːtərəʊ]	ureterography [jʊəˌriːtəˈrɒgrəfɪ] ureterolithotomy [jʊəˌriːtərəlɪˈθɒtəmɪ] ureterostenosis [jʊəˌriːtərəsteˈnəʊsɪs]		
urethra			
urethr(o) [jʊəˈriːθrəʊ]	urethralgia [ˌjʊəriˈθrældʒɪə] urethrorrhagia [jʊəˌriːθrɒˈreɪdʒɪə] urethroscopy [ˌjʊərəˈθrɒskəpɪ]		
meatus, passageway			
meat(o) [ˈmiːətəʊ]	meatoscopy [ˌmiːəˈtɒskəpɪ] meatotomy [ˌmiːəˈtɒtəmɪ]		
urinary bladder, sac			
cyst(o) [ˈsɪstəʊ]	cystitis [sɪsˈtaɪtɪs] cystocele [ˈsɪstəsiːl] cholecystectomy [ˌkɒlɪsɪsˈtektəmɪ]	-cele=swelling	
vesic(o) [ˈvesɪkəʊ]	vesicocele [ˈvesɪkəˌsiːl] vesiculitis [vɪˌsɪkjʊˈlaɪtɪs] vesiculotomy [vɪˌsɪkjʊˈlɒtəmɪ]		
kidney			

(to be continued)

ren(o) ['renəʊ]	circumrenal [sɜːkʌm'riːnəl] renculus ['renkjʊləs] renopathy [re'nɒpəθɪ]	circum-=around or encircling	
nephr(o) ['nefrəʊ]	nephrolith ['nefrəlɪθ] nephrology [ne'frɒlədʒɪ] nephrorrhagia [ˌnefrəʊ'reɪdʒɪə]		
ball			
glomer(o) [gləʊ'merəʊ]	glomerular [gləʊ'merjʊlə] glomerulitis [glɒˌmerjʊ'laɪtɪs] glomerulonephritis [gləʊˌmerjʊləʊne'fraɪtɪs]		
renal pelvis			
pyel(o) ['paɪələʊ]	pyelonephritis [ˌpaɪələʊne'fraɪtɪs] pyelolithotomy [ˌpaɪələʊlɪ'θɒtəmɪ] pyelogram ['paɪələgræm]		
cortex			
cortic(o) ['kɔːtɪkəʊ]	adrenocorticotropin [əˌdriːnəʊˌkɔːtɪkəʊ'trɒpɪn] corticosteroid [ˌkɔːtɪkəʊ'sterɔɪd] cortisol ['kɔːtɪsɒl]	adren(o)=adrenal glands	
medulla			
medull(o) [me'dʌləʊ]	medullary [me'dʌlərɪ] medullectomy [ˌmedʌ'lektəmɪ]		
calcium			
calc(o) ['kælkəʊ] calci(o) ['kælsɪəʊ]	calcitonin [ˌkælsɪ'təʊnɪn] calcinosis [ˌkælsɪ'nəʊsɪs] hypercalcemia [ˌhaɪpəkæl'siːmɪə]		

(to be continued)

stone, calculus			
lith(o) [ˈlɪθəʊ]	lithotripsy [ˈlɪθəˌtrɪpsi] lithogenesis [ˌlɪθəʊˈdʒenɪsɪs] lithotomy [lɪˈθɒtəmɪ]		
nitrogen			
azo [ˈæzəʊ] azot(o) [ˈæzəʊtəʊ]	azomycin [ˌæzəʊˈmaɪsɪn] azotemia [ˌæzəʊˈtiːmɪə] hypazoturia [haɪpəzəʊˈtjuːrɪə]		
pus			
py(o) [paɪəʊ]	pyogenesis [ˌpaɪəʊˈdʒenɪsɪs] pyorrhea [ˌpaɪəˈriːə] pyuria [paɪˈjʊərɪə]	-genesis=origin, formation	
night			
noct(o) [ˈnɒktəʊ] nocti [ˈnɒkti]	nocturia [nɒkˈtjʊərɪə] nocturnal [nɒkˈtɜːnl]		
scanty, little, few, less than normal			
olig(o) [ˈɒlɪgəʊ]	oligotrophy [ˌɒlɪˈgɒtrəfi] oligomenorrhea [ˌɒlɪgəʊˌmenɜːˈriːə] oliguria [ˌɒlɪˈgjʊərɪə]	-trophy=nutrition, growth	
many, much			
poly [ˈpɒli]	polymyositis [ˌpɒlɪˌmaɪəˈsaɪtɪs] polyphagia [ˌpɒlɪˈfeɪdʒɪə] polydipsia [ˌpɒlɪˈdɪpsɪə]	phag(o)=eating	
downward displacement or dropping			
ptos [ˈtəʊs]	gastroptosis [ˌgæstrɒpˈtəʊsɪs] nephroptosis [ˌnefrɒpˈtəʊsɪs]		

(to be continued)

fix, fasten			
pex [ˈpeks]	nephropexy [ˈnefrəˌpeksɪ] hysteropexy [ˈhɪstərəpeksɪ]	hyster(o)=uterus	
ketone			
ket(o) [ˈki:təʊ]	ketosteroid [kɪtəʊˈsterɔɪd] ketosis [kɪˈtəʊsɪs] ketoacidosis [ˌki:təʊˌæsɪˈdəʊsɪs]		
albumin (a protein in the blood)			
albumin(o) [ˈælbjʊmɪnəʊ]	albuminuria [ˌælbjʊmɪˈnjʊərɪə] albuminemia [ˌælbjʊmɪˈni:mɪə] albuminoid [ælˈbju:mɪˌnɔɪd]		

Vocabulary Study

Task 1

Directions: *Match each of the following terms with its definition and underline the strong part of each word where there are two or more syllables.*

(1) meatotomy	A. X-ray examination of the ureter after injection of a contrast medium
(2) ureterography	B. pertaining to or of a renal glomerulus
(3) cystitis	C. an inflammation of the urethra
(4) urethritis	D. an incision made to enlarge a meatus of the urethra or ureter
(5) glomerular	E. inflammation of the urinary bladder

(6) lithogenesis	A. hemorrhage from the kidney
(7) pyogenesis	B. abnormally excessive urination during the night
(8) nocturia	C. formation of pus
(9) polydipsia	D. formation of calculi, or stones
(10) nephrorrhagia	E. excessive thirst

Task 2

Directions: Fill in the blanks with appropriate words for body parts.

(1) Cystoscope is an instrument for examining the interior of the _____.

(2) Urethralgia is the pain in the _____.

(3) Pyelogram is a radiograph or series of radiographs of the _____ and ureter, following injection of contrast medium.

(4) Adrenocorticotropin is a hormone secreted by the anterior lobe of the pituitary gland that stimulates the cortex of the _____ to secrete its hormones, including corticosterone.

(5) Nephroptosis refers to the medical condition in which the _____ does not remain fixed in its proper location but has abnormal mobility.

(6) Pyelonephritis is an inflammation of the kidney and upper _____ that usually results from noncontagious bacterial infection of the bladder.

(7) Meatoscopy is the visual examination of a/an _____, especially that of the urethra.

(8) Calicotomy refers to the incision of a/an _____.

(9) A person with polycystic kidney disease has a hereditary condition in which the kidneys are enlarged and contain many _____.

(10) Glomerulitis is the inflammation of a/an _____.

Task 3

Directions: Write a word for the following definitions using the word parts provided.

medull(o)	urethr(o)	adren(o)	circum-	-rrhagia
-al	vesic(o)	-cele	-scopy	ren(o)

(1) visual inspection of the urethra _____

(2) pertaining to the medulla of the adrenal gland _____

(3) hernia of the urinary bladder _____

(4) urethral bleeding _____

(5) surrounding the kidney in whole or part _____

meat(o)	ur(o)	cyst(o)	-tomy	calc(o)
-ology	-ectomy	-emia	hyper-	chol(o)

(6) toxic condition resulting from kidney disease _____

(7) an incision made to enlarge a meatus _____

(8) surgical removal of the gallbladder _____

(9) the medical specialty concerned with the urinary system _____

(10) high level of calcium in the blood _____

lith(o)	nephr(o)	py(o)	-trophy	-pexy
-rrhea	olig(o)	-tripsy	hyster(o)	-itis

(11) deficient nutrition _____

(12) inflammation of the kidney _____

(13) crushing of a stone _____

(14) a discharge of pus _____

(15) fixation of a displaced uterus by surgery _____

Case Study 7-1

Renal Calculi

A.A., a 48-year-old woman, was admitted to the inpatient unit from the ER with severe right flank pain unresponsive to analgesics. Her pain did not decrease with administration of 100 mg of IV meperidine. She had a three-month history of chronic UTI. Six months ago, she had been prescribed calcium supplements for low bone density. Her gynecologist warned her that calcium could be a problem for people who are "stone formers". A.A. was unaware that she might be at risk. An IV urogram showed a right staghorn calculus. The diagnosis was further confirmed by a renal ultrasound. A renal flow scan showed normal perfusion and no obstruction. Kidney function was 37 percent on the right and 63 percent on the left. The pain became intermittent, and A.A. had no hematuria, dysuria, frequency, urgency, or nocturia. Urinalysis revealed no albumin, glucose, bacteria, or blood; there was evidence of cells, crystals, and casts.

A.A. was transferred to surgery for a cystoscopic ureteral laser lithotripsy, insertion of a right retrograde ureteral catheter, and right percutaneous nephrolithotomy. A ureteral calculus was fragmented with a pulsed-dye laser. Most of the staghorn was removed from the renal pelvis with no remaining stone in the renal calices. She was discharged two days later and ordered to strain her urine for evidence of stones for the next week .

Task 4

Directions: *Select the best answer based on the information provided in the case of Renal Calculi.*

(1) Which is NOT the reason why the woman was admitted to the inpatient unit?

 A. She got severe right flank pain.

 B. She had a three-month history of chronic UTI.

 C. Her pain was not responsive to analgesics.

 D. Her pain did not reduce with administration of meperidine.

(2) Which of the following could NOT be about the patient's medical history?

 A. She had a three-month history of chronic urinary tract infection.

 B. Calcium supplements had been prescribed for her low bone density.

 C. She might be at risk of "stone formers".

 D. Kidney function was 37 percent on the right and 63 percent on the left.

(3) The term "percutaneous" means _____.

 A. under the skin   B. through the skin

 C. on the surface   D. with a catheter

(4) The abbreviation IV means _____ in the case.

 A. independent variable   B. intravenous injection

 C. initial velocity   D. inverted vertical

(5) Meperidine refers to a type of drug which is _____.

 A. analgesic   B. antibiotics

 C. placebo   D. antidepressant

(6) The following diagnostic tests were performed EXCEPT _____.

 A. IV urogram   B. ultrasound

 C. renal flow scan   D. urine culture

(7) The term "perfusion" means_____.

 A. size   B. shape

 C. passage of fluid   D. surrounding tissue

(8) What was the woman's pain like?

 A. Dull pain.   B. Persistent pain.

 C. Coming and going pain.   D. Acute pain.

(9) Which of the following is NOT true about urinalysis?

 A. There is no proteinin the urine.

 B. There is no crystals in the urine.

 C. There is no glucose in the urine.

 D. There is no bacteria or blood in the urine.

(10) Which of the following is TRUE about the diagnosis of the woman?

A. Staghorn calculus.　　　　　B. Blood in the urine.

C. Difficult urination.　　　　　D. Excessive urination at night.

Case Study 7-2

Artificial Urinary Sphincter Implantation

An 81-year-old male was hospitalized at the Urology ward due to severe urinary incontinence from mixed causes with clear stress-related elements. The urethral dysfunction occurred about 1 year ago following the endoscopic cervico-urethral disobstruction operation carried out in another facility. It has to be reported that in July 1993 a surgical operation was carried out in order to correct the sphincteric dysfunction according to Lenzi's method that provides for a sinking of the urethra in the corpus cavernosum. Despite from this therapeutic attempt, the patient kept showing a severe urinary incontinence mostly orthostatic. Treatment consisted of a conservative therapy with anticholinergic drugs and of a perineal electrostimulation without achieving any appreciable result.

Therefore, hospitalization was carried out during which the patient underwent the case evaluations in order to confirm the possibility of an artificial sphincter implantation. Such evaluations gave evidence of a high excretory duct within normal limits; the bladder showed normal capacity in the absence of refluxes and mainly in the absence of residual intravesical obstructions with a complete reservoir emptying.

The patient, therefore, underwent surgical operation of Scott's AMS 800 artificial urinary sphincter implantation at the urethral bulb (4.5 cm cuff; 61—70 cm water balloon; osmolarity of 343 milliosmoles/liter). The postsurgical course was normal except for a small hematoma in the scrotal pump that, however, did not bring about a sphincter inflammation. As the follow-up examination carried out the patient confirmed a perfect continence with good flow and a prosthesis activity which

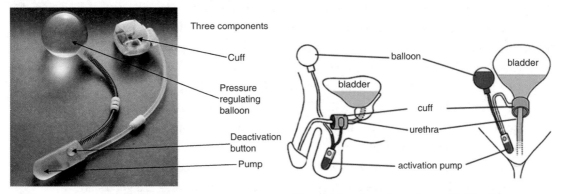

Figure 1 AMS 800 artificial urinary sphincter

Figure 2 Implantation of an artificial sphincter to a man (left) and a woman (right)

appeared to be normal. The patient had to compress the pump only once and apparently a good filling of the cuff was reached after miction. On the same occasion a uroflowmetry was carried out. It showed a maximum urinary flow 42mL/sec with absent echograph residue. The two renal parenchymas appeared to be normal without any pyelo-ureteral dilatation.

Task 5

Directions: *Complete the following notes of the case report.*

Sex: _____   Age: _____

Diagnosis: _____

Case history: _____

_____

_____

_____

Treatment: _____

Evaluation before surgery: _____

Postsurgical course: _____

_____

Medical Term Extension

The Metric System

Introduction

In the United States, both the U.S. customary measurement system and the metric system are used, especially in medical, scientific, and technical fields. In most other countries, the metric system is the primary system of measurement. If you travel to other countries, you will see that road signs list distances in kilometers and milk is sold in liters. People in many countries use words like "kilometer," "liter," and "milligram" to measure the length, volume, and weight of different objects. These measurement units are part of the metric system.

Unlike the U.S. customary system of measurement, the metric system is based on 10s. For example, a liter is 10 times larger than a deciliter, and a centigram is 10 times larger than a milligram. This idea of "10" is not present in the U.S. customary system—there are 12 inches in a foot, and 3 feet in a yard…and 5,280 feet in a mile!

So, what if you have to find out how many milligrams are in a decigram? Or, what if you want to convert meters to kilometers? Understanding how the metric system works is a good start.

What is Metric?

The metric system uses units such as meter, liter, and gram to measure length, liquid volume, and mass, just as the U.S. customary system uses feet, quarts, and ounces to measure these.

In addition to the difference in the basic units, the metric system is based on 10s, and different measures for length include kilometer, meter, decimeter, centimeter, and millimeter. Notice that the word "meter" is part of all of these units.

The metric system also applies the idea that units within the system get larger or smaller by a power of 10. This means that a meter is 100 times larger than a centimeter, and a kilogram is 1,000 times heavier than a gram. You will explore this idea a bit later. For now, notice how this idea of "getting bigger or smaller by 10" is very different than the relationship between units in the U.S. customary system, where 3 feet equals 1 yard, and 16 ounces equals 1 pound.

Length, Mass, and Volume

The table below shows the basic units of the metric system. Note that the names of all metric units follow from these three basic units.

Length	Mass	Volume
basic units		
meter	gram	liter
other units you may see		
kilometer	kilogram	dekaliter
centimeter	centigram	centiliter
millimeter	milligram	milliliter

In the metric system, the basic unit of length is the meter. A meter is slightly larger than a yardstick, or just over three feet.

The basic metric unit of mass is the gram. A regular-sized paperclip has a mass of about 1 gram.

Among scientists, one gram is defined as the mass of water that would fill a 1-centimeter cube. You may notice that the word "mass" is used here instead of "weight". In the sciences and technical fields, a distinction is made between weight and mass. Weight is a measure of the pull of gravity on an object. For this reason, an object's weight would be different if it was weighed on Earth or on the moon because of the difference in the gravitational forces. However, the object's mass would remain the same in both places because mass measures the amount of substance in an object. As long as you are planning on only measuring objects on Earth, you can use mass/weight fairly interchangeably—but it is worth noting that there is a difference!

Finally, the basic metric unit of volume is the liter. A liter is slightly larger than a quart.

Task 6

Directions: *Study the metric conversion chart, and then fill in the tables.*

Metric Conversion Chart

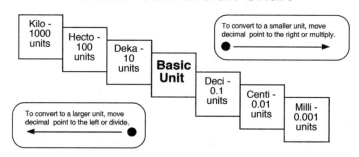

Units of length		Units of weight		Units of volume	
Full form	Unit abbreviation	Full form	Unit abbreviation	Full form	Unit abbreviation
kilometer			kg		kl
hectometer		hectogram			hl
decameter			dag		dal
meter		gram			l
decimeter			dg		dl
centimeter		centigram			cl
millimeter			mg		ml

Unit abbreviation	Full form
g/L	
L/L	
×10^9/L	
mmol/L	
umol/L or μmol/L	
U/L	

Task 7

Directions: *Circle the recommended abbreviation for the metric units of measurement.*

(1) grams

    A. gr   B. gms   C. G   D. g

(2) milligrams

    A. mgm   B. mg   C. Mgs   D. mcg

(3) liters

    A. L   B. l   C. ls   D. Ls

(4) milliliters

 A. m   B. mL   C. mg   D. mLs

(5) microgram

 A. μg   B. mg   C. mcg   D. mc

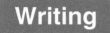

Writing

Good Versus Poor Scientific Writing: An Orientation

"Everything that can be thought at all
can be thought clearly. Everything that can be said can be said clearly."
Ludwig Wittgenstein

Good scientific writing hinges on the ability to express complicated concepts in clear words, thus pointing out the beauty of science without unnecessary decoration. Although we would all agree that the beauty of science is in the science itself, not in the language used to describe it, we have to accept that a confusing account of our findings will not do justice to the science that lies behind it.

What can we, as writers, do to ensure that our scientific message reaches the intended target population?

Good scientific writing is

• *understandable:* Readers should read our paper in full, rather than discarding it after a few sentences because the text makes no sense to them. We should also bear in mind that while the international scientific language is English, the native tongue of readers (other scientists, regulators, etc.) may be a language other than English.

• *transparent:* The written report is often the only way for readers to access the research done. Thus, our scientific paper is the only "window" through which readers can view our "laboratory".

• *clear:* Some scientists inadvertently keep their acquired knowledge to themselves rather than share it with the scientific community or their peers. They may write in a vague, complicated, and unstructured manner, using ample ornamentation that distracts the reader. However, good scientific writing should inform rather than confuse the readers.

• *credible:* As scientists, we have to be credible to gain our readers' respect. For instance, if we apply for a research grant, our written proposal must be convincing, both in terms of the concepts and the language used to describe them. Similarly, a paper written in an accurate, compelling, and logical style conveys to the readers that the research described was also done accordingly. The way we express ourselves portrays the way we think.

• *efficient:* By improving our scientific writing skills, we essentially gain time. Poorly written papers may be delayed or even rejected although the science behind them may be of considerable interest. A reputation of being a good and reliable scientific writer will open doors to more publishing and positive feedback.

• *simple:* Text devoid of unnecessary decorative words is more readily understood than complicated, ornamental expositions.

When we declare that a certain text is better than another, we rely on a scale of values, with "good" at one end and "poor" at the other. But who sets the standards for "good" and "poor" scientific writing? Who is the ultimate judge? Who censors the quality of our scientific texts? While general opinion of what is "correct" may be divided, there are certain bodies or sources that we usually accept as authorities. These include dictionaries, grammarians, linguists, editors, and teachers, scientific community, set traditions and accepted trends.

The ultimate judgment of the quality of our scientific writing efforts lies with the readers themselves. We have conventions to follow, guidelines to adhere to, and trends to observe. When evaluating the "power" of a scientific manuscript—your own or some other author's—you may find it helpful to consult the document standards listed in Table 1.

Table 1 Document standards

Standard	Description
Purpose	The purpose and objectives of the study must be obvious and unambiguous.
Conformity	Text has to conform to given formats and style requirements.
Accuracy	The wording must be grammatically correct, concise, and precise. All information and data provided must be accurate.
Consistency	Terminology should be consistent and appropriate. Only commonly known abbreviations should be used, and these must be used consistently.
Logic and flow	The manuscript should be a "story" with a clear message based on a logical train of thought.
Context	New findings must be reported and interpreted in the context of findings already published and must be congruent with accepted institutional or regulatory values.
Structure	A logical structure (i.e., headings and subheadings, paragraphs, and data displays) should be chosen. A well-balanced mixture of text and visuals (e.g., figures and tables) should be chosen, in line with the relevant instructions for authors.
Data presentation	High-quality data should be presented clearly, using tables and figures as appropriate. Duplication of data displays must be avoided.

Clearly, adherence to the rules of grammar and spelling, as well as the use of the appropriate terminology in the relevant scientific field, must be considered "base-line". In other words, we owe it to the ethics of writing to observe the fundamentals of proper communication, particularly if we communicate in writing. Misspelled words not only confuse—they often annoy the readers to the extent they no longer wish to read the full text. Moreover, poor grammar and erroneous use of technical or scientific terms will jeopardize the credibility of our results. By extrapolation, it is our credibility as scientists that is at stake.

It is important to realize that there is, in fact, room for personal opinion even in the context of scientific writing. This implies that certain issues are not simply "correct" or "incorrect". A particular word may be preferred over another, but the less preferable term may not be wrong as such. Let us consider the following sentences:

- In this study, we took blood samples immediately before starting the infusion.

- In this study, we took blood samples immediately prior to starting the infusion.

Is "before" or "prior to" correct here? Clearly, both terms are correct, and the choice solely depends on your personal preference. American writers may go for "prior to", while European writers may favor the more commonly used "before". The same applies to terms such as "following" and "after". Again, the two terms can be used interchangeably in principle, but my advice is to use "after" instead of "following" for two reasons, i.e., the term "after" is shorter, and "following" is used far too often in scientific writing because of its various meanings.

In conclusion, we should always keep in mind that excessive arguing about the "rights" and "wrongs" of scientific writing is a poor investment of precious time, especially if the issue is simply a question of personal opinion.

Task 1

Directions: *The following will be groups of extracts of EMP writing. Decide which version in each group is better than the other, and explain why.*

Group 1
→ The patient's hemoglobin was normal.
→ The patient's hemoglobin levels were normal.
→ **Comment:**

___

Group 2
→ The throat culture was negative.
→ The throat culture was negative for β-hemolytic streptococci（溶血性链球菌）.
→ **Comment:**

___

Group 3
→ The physical examination was normal.
→ The results of the physical examination were normal.
→ **Comment:**

___

Group 4
→ The electrocardiogram was negative.
→ The electrocardiogram showed abnormalities in the alpha wave activity.
→ **Comment:**

Group 5

→ By using antidepressants, we were able to treat the patient effectively.

→ We were able to treat the patient effectively by administering antidepressants.

→ **Comment:**

Group 6

→ No bacteria were observed using dimethyl sulfoxide as a solvent.

→ When dimethyl sulfoxide was used as a solvent, no bacteria were observed.

→ With dimethyl sulfoxide as a solvent, no bacteria were observed.

→ **Comment:**

Group 7

→ A patient may have a fever of 39.5℃ .

→ A patient may have a temperature of 39.5℃ .

→ **Comment:**

Group 8

→ The postoperative mortality rate was 10.1% (9 patients), and the overall 5-year survival was 25%, respectively.

→ The postoperative mortality rate and the overall 5-year survival were 10.1% (9 patients) and 25%, respectively.

→ **Comment:**

Group 9

→ The patient was a 55-year-old female with a history of fainting. The attending physician performed a physical examination and ordered laboratory testing. She had high levels of blood glucose and hypercholesterolemia.

→ The patient was a 55-year-old female with a history of fainting. A physical examination and laboratory testing were performed at admission. Blood screening revealed hypercholesterolemia. High levels of blood glucose were also noted. She was admitted to our department for further testing.

→ **Comment:**

Group 10

→ In light of the previous trial's results, the levels detected in our study are relatively higher.

→ In light of the previous trial's results, the levels detected in our study are higher. / In light of the previous trial's results, the levels detected in our study are relatively high.

→ **Comment:**

Group 11

→ The efficacy of ATO has been attributed to the induction of apoptosis, inhibiting proliferation and angiogenesis, and promotion of differentiation.

→ The efficacy of ATO has been attributed to the induction of apoptosis, inhibition of proliferation and angiogenesis, and promotion of differentiation.

→ **Comment:**

Group 12

→ This method is labor intensive, time consuming, expensive, and relies upon the submission of fresh material to the diagnostic laboratory.

→ This method is labor intensive, time consuming, and expensive, and it relies upon the submission of fresh material to the diagnostic laboratory.

→ **Comment:**

Group 13

→ These symptoms are associated with aging, cancer and other diseases.

→ These symptoms are associated with aging and with cancer and other diseases.

→ **Comment:**

Group 14

→ Additional work was needed to find other materials that are readily available, cost effective and that demonstrate comparable catalytic effects for the tri-iodide reduction in DSSCs.

→ Additional work was needed to find other materials that are readily available and cost effective and that demonstrate comparable catalytic effects for the tri-iodide reduction in DSSCs.

→ **Comment:**

Group 15

→ Our results suggest that Protein X might catalyze a reverse reaction.

→ Our results suggest that Protein X catalyzes a reverse reaction.

→ **Comment:**

Group 16

→ These new compounds may potentially reduce the side effects of current treatments.

→ These new compounds have the potential to reduce the side effects of current treatments.

→ **Comment:**

Group 17

→ The existence of degradation products implies that contaminating proteins appear to be present.

→ The existence of degradation products implies the presence of contaminating proteins.

→ **Comment:**

Group 18

→ These four genes are possible candidates for knockdown to reduce Protein X levels.

→ These four genes are candidates for knockdown to reduce Protein X levels.

→ **Comment:**

Group 19

→ The positive control exhibited an increase of 14%, the negative control exhibited an increase of 3%, and the experimental group exhibited an increase of 16%.

→ The positive control exhibited an increase of 14%; the negative control, 0%; and the experimental group, 16%.

→ **Comment:**

Group 20

→ The positive control exhibited an increase of 14%, and the negative control exhibited an increase of 0%.

→ The positive control exhibited an increase of 14%; the negative control, 0%.

→ **Comment:**

Group 21

→ The positive control grew by 4 cm, and the negative control grew by 1 cm.

→ The positive control grew by 4 cm, and the negative control by 1 cm.

→ **Comment:**

Group 22

→ The positive control exhibited an increase, and the negative control did not exhibit an increase.

→ The positive control exhibited an increase, and the negative control did not.

→ **Comment:**

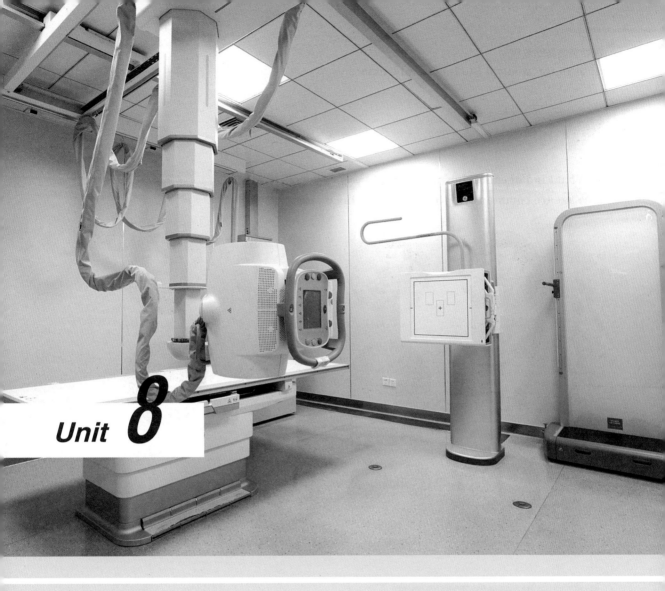

Unit 8

The Endocrine System

√ 听力音频
√ 听力文本
√ 课件资源

Warm-up

1. What kind of endocrine problems did you ever experience?
2. What are common symptoms of endocrine diseases?

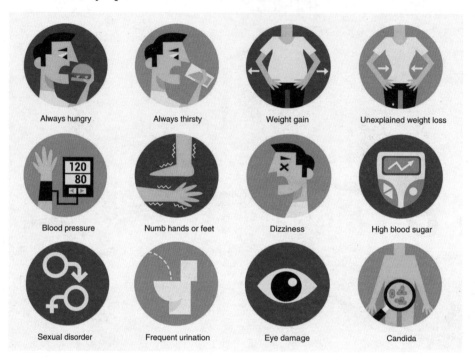

Theme Reading

Homeostasis depends on the precise regulation of the organs and organ systems of the body. The nervous and endocrine systems are two major systems responsible for that regulation. Together they regulate and coordinate the activity of nearly all other body structures.The endocrine system is an information signaling system much like the nervous system. However, the nervous system uses nerves to conduct information, whereas the endocrine system uses blood vessels as information channels.

The Endocrine System

Objectives

☆ *List the glands that make up the endocrine system.*
☆ *State the location of each endocrine gland in the body.*
☆ *Name the hormones secreted by each endocrine gland and their functions.*

A gland is any organ that produces a secretion. Endocrine glands (Figure 8-1), also called ductless glands, are organized groups of tissues which use materials from the blood or lymph to make new compounds called hormones. The products of the endocrine glands were named hormones (Gk. Horman, to urge on, to stir up) because those first discovered had the effect of stimulating physiologic action. The name is not entirely suitable because some hormones "depress" rather than "excite", and others still have other functions. Although produced in extremely small quantities—"trace" amounts—they have remarkable effects in the regulation of bodily functions.

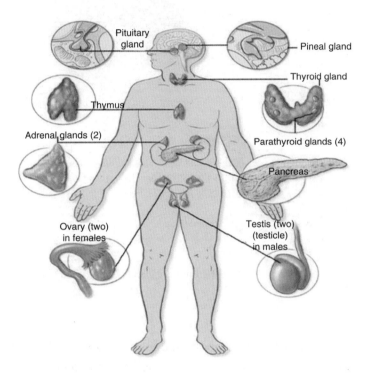

Figure 8-1 The endocrine system

There is another type of gland called an exocrine gland, in which the secretions from the gland must go through a duct. This duct then carries the secretion to a body surface or organ. Exocrine glands include the sweat gland, the salivary glands, the **lacrimal** gland, and the pancreas. In fact, the pancreas performs both as an exocrine gland and an endocrine gland.

Pituitary Gland

The pituitary gland, also called the **hypophysis**, is a small gland about the size of a pea. It is located at the base of the brain within the **sella turcica**, a small bony depression in the **sphenoid bone** inferior to the **hypothalamus** of the brain. The hypothalamus is an important autonomic nervous system and endocrine control center of the brain located inferior to the thalamus. The pituitary gland is connected to the hypothalamus by a stalk called the **infundibulum**. The pituitary is divided into two lobes: the larger anterior pituitary lobe is made up of epithelial cells; the smaller posterior pituitary lobe consists primarily of nerve fibers and **neuroglial** cells that support the nerve fibers. The pituitary gland is known as the master gland of the body because of its major influence on the body's activities, such as growth, kidney function, birth, milk production, etc.

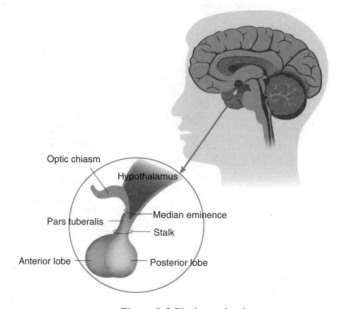

Figure 8-2 Pituitary gland

Anterior Pituitary Lobe

The anterior pituitary lobe secretes six hormones. Growth hormone (GH), also called **somatotropin**, stimulates the growth of bones, muscles, and other organs by increasing protein synthesis. It also resists protein breakdown during periods of food deprivation and favors fat breakdown. **Prolactin** hormone (PRL) helps promote development of the breast during pregnancy and stimulates the production of milk after childbirth. The function in males is unknown. Thyroid-stimulating hormone (TSH), also called **thyrotropin**, stimulates the growth and secretion of the thyroid gland. **Adrenocorticotropic** hormone (ACTH), also called **corticotropin**, stimulates the growth and secretion of the adrenal cortex. ACTH increases the secretion of a hormone from the adrenal cortex called **cortisol**, or **hydrocortisone**, and ACTH is required to keep the adrenal cortex from degenerating. ACTH molecules also bind to **melanocytes** in the skin and increase skin **pigmentation**. **Follicle**-stimulating hormone (FSH) stimulates the growth of the **graafian follicle** and the production of **estrogen** in females, and stimulates the production of sperm in males. **Luteinizing hormone** (LH) stimulates the growth of the graafian follicle, the production of estrogen and the formation of the **corpus luteum** after **ovulation**, which produces **progesterone** in the female. In males, LH stimulates the secretion of the sex hormone **testosterone** from the testes. It is sometimes called the **interstitial** cell-stimulating hormone (ICSH) because it stimulates interstitial cells of the testes to secrete testosterone.

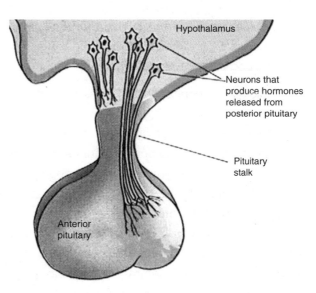

Figure 8-3 Anterior pituitary lobe

Posterior Pituitary Lobe

The hormones produced by the hypothalamus are stored in the posterior pituitary lobe. Antidiuretic hormone (ADH) is also called vasopressin.The name vasopressin may lead to confusion because it causes little or no vasoconstriction. ADH maintains the water balance by increasing the absorption of water in the kidney tubules. Sometimes drugs called diuretics are used to inhibit the action of ADH. The result is an increase in urinary output and a decrease in blood volume, thus decreasing blood pressure.

Oxytocin is released during childbirth, causing strong contractions of the uterus and milk ejection, or milk "let-down", from the breasts in lactating women. Commercial preparations of oxytocin are given under certain conditions to assist in childbirth and to constrict **uterine** blood vessels following childbirth.

Thyroid Gland

The thyroid gland is a butterfly-shaped mass of tissue located in the anterior part of the neck. It lies on either side of the larynx over the trachea. Its general shape is that of the letter H. It is about 2 inches long with two lobes joined by strands of thyroid tissue called the isthmus. In place of the **isthmus** there is often a pyramidal

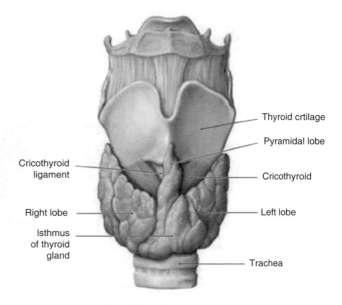

Figure 8-4 Thyroid gland

lobe, whose apex points cranially to the embryonic origin of the thyroid at the base of the tongue. The thyroid gland has a rich blood supply. In fact, it has been estimated that about 4 to 5 liters of blood pass through the gland every hour.

The thyroid gland secretes three hormones: **thyroxine**, **triiodothyronine** and **calcitonin**. The first two are iodine-bearing derivatives of the **amino acid**, **tyrosine**. Triiodothyronine is 5 to 10 times more active than thyroxine, but its activity is less prolonged. However, the two have the same effect and both hormones are produced by the follicle cells of the thyroid gland. The functions of thyroxin (T_4) and triiodothyronine (T_3) are as follows: (1) controls the rate of metabolism in the body; (2) stimulates protein synthesis and thus helps tissue growth; (3) stimulates the breakdown of liver **glycogen** to glucose. The thyroid-stimulating hormone (TSH) controls the production and secretion of the thyroid hormones from the thyroid gland. Calcitonin is another hormone produced and secreted by the thyroid gland. It controls the calcium ion concentration in the body by maintaining a proper calcium level in the bloodstream. The constant level of calcium in the blood and tissues is maintained by the action of calcitonin and **parathormone**.

Parathyroid Glands

The parathyroid glands are tiny glands attached to the posterior surface of the thyroid gland. They secrete the hormone parathormone, which also controls the concentration of calcium in the bloodstream. Parathormone stimulates an increase in the number and size of specialized bone cells referred to as **osteoclasts**. Osteoclasts quickly invade hard bone tissue, digesting large amounts of the bony material containing calcium. As this process continues, calcium leaves the bone and is released into the bloodstream, increasing the calcium blood level. Thus, parathormone and calcitonin have opposite, or **antagonistic**, effects to one another.

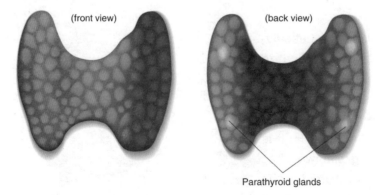

Figure 8-5 Parathyroid glands

Adrenal Glands

The two adrenal glands are located on top of each kidney. Each gland has two parts: the cortex and the medulla. **Adrenocorticotropic** hormone (ACTH) from the pituitary glands stimulates the activity of the cortex of the adrenal gland. The hormones secreted by the adrenal cortex are known as corticoids. The **corticoids** are very effective as anti-inflammatory drugs.

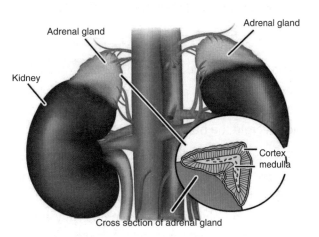

Figure 8-6 Adrenal glands

The cortex secretes three groups of corticoids, each of which is of great importance. **Mineralocorticoids**—mainly **aldosterone**, affect the kidney tubules by speeding up the reabsorption of sodium into the blood circulation and increasing the excretion of **potassium** from the blood. They also speed up the reabsorption of water by the kidneys. Aldosterone is used in the treatment of Addison's disease to replace deficient secretion of mineralocorticoids.

Glucocorticoids—namely **cortisone** and cortisol—increase the amount of glucose in the blood. This is done by the conversion of proteins and fats to glycogen in the liver, followed by breakdown of the glycogen into glucose. These glucocorticoids also help the body resist the aggravations caused by various everyday stresses. In addition, these hormones seem to decrease edema in inflammation and reduce pain by inhibiting pain-causing **prostaglandin**.

The third class of hormones secreted by the adrenal cortex is the **androgens**. They are able to stimulate the development of male sexual characteristics. Small amounts of androgens are secreted from the adrenal cortex in both males and females. In adult males, most androgens are secreted by the **testes**. In adult females, the adrenal androgen influences the female sex drive. If the secretion of sex hormones from the adrenal cortex is abnormally high, exaggerated male characteristics develop in both males and females. This condition is most apparent in females and males before puberty when the effects are not masked by the secretion of androgen by the testes.

The medulla of the adrenal gland secretes **epinephrine** and **norepinephrine**. Epinephrine, or adrenalin, is a powerful cardiac stimulant. It functions by bringing about a release of more glucose from stored glycogen or muscle activity and increasing the force and rate of the heartbeat. This chemical activity increases cardiac output and venous return and raises the **systolic** blood pressure. The adrenal medulla responds to the **sympathetic** nervous system. Epinephrine and norepinephrine are referred to as the fight-or-flight hormones because of their role in preparing the body for vigorous physical activity.

Pancreas

The pancreas is located behind the stomach and performs both as an exocrine gland and an endocrine gland. The pancreas produces pancreatic juices which go through a duct into the small intestines and it also has a special group of cells known as **islets of Langerhans** which secrete the hormone **insulin** directly into the bloodstream.

The islet cells are distributed throughout the pancreas. These cells were named the islets of Langerhans after the doctor who discovered them. Beta cells produce insulin, which (1) promotes the utilization of glucose in the cells, necessary for the maintenance of normal levels of blood glucose; (2) promotes fatty acid transport and fat deposition into cells; (3) promotes amino acid transport into cells; and (4) facilitates protein synthesis. Lack of insulin secretion by the islet cells causes diabetes mellitus.

The alpha cells contained in the islets of Langerhans secrete the hormone glucagon. The action of **glucagon** may be antagonistic or opposite to that of insulin. Glucagon's function is to increase the level of glucose in the bloodstream. This is done by stimulating the conversion of liver glycogen to glucose. The control of glucagon secretion is achieved by negative feedback. Low glucose levels in the bloodstream stimulate the alpha cells to secrete glucagon, which quickly increases the glucose level in the bloodstream.

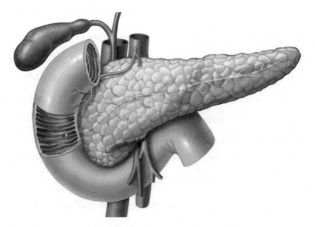

Figure 8-7 Pancreas

Vocabulary

adrenocorticotropic [əˌdriːnəʊˌkɔːtəkəʊˈtrɒpɪk]　acting on or stimulating the adrenal cortex

aldosterone [ælˈdɒstəˌrəʊn]　a hormone produced by the adrenal cortex, instrumental in the regulation of sodium and potassium reabsorption by the cells of the tubular portion of the kidney

amino acid [əˈmiːnəʊ] [ˈæsɪd]　organic compounds containing an amino group and a carboxylic acid group

androgen [ˈændrədʒən]　any substance, as testosterone or androsterone, that promotes male characteristics

antagonistic [ænˌtægəˈnɪstɪk]　marked by or resulting from antagonism

calcitonin [ˌkælsɪˈtəʊnɪn]　a hormone secreted by the thyroid that inhibits the release of calcium from the skeleton and prevents a build-up of calcium in the blood

corpus luteum [ˈkɔːpəs] [ljuːˈtiːəm]　a yellow glandular mass of tissue that forms in a Graafian follicle following release of an ovum

corticoid [ˈkɔːtɪˌkɔɪd]　any steroid hormone produced by the adrenal cortex that affects carbohydrate, protein, and electrolyte metabolism, gonad function, and immune response

corticotropin [kɔːtɪkəʊˈtrəʊpən]　a hormone of the anterior pituitary that stimulates the production of steroids in the cortex of the adrenal glands

epinephrine [ˌepɪˈnefrɪn]　also called adrenaline, the principal blood-pressure raising hormone secreted by the adrenal medulla and is used medicinally especially as a heart stimulant, a vasoconstrictor in controlling hemorrhages of the skin, and a muscle relaxant in bronchial asthma

estrogen [ˈestrədʒən]　any of several major female sex hormones produced primarily by ovarian follicles, capable of inducing estrus, producing secondary female sex characteristics, and preparing the uterus for the reception of a fertilized

follicle [ˈfɒlɪkəl]　a small anatomical cavity or deep narrow-mouthed depression; a vesicle in the mammalian ovary that contains a developing egg surrounded by a covering of cells

glucagon [ˈgluːkəˌgən]　a hormone secreted by the pancreas that acts in opposition to insulin in the regulation of blood glucose levels

glucocorticoid [ˌgluːkəʊˈkɔːtɪˌkɔɪd]　any of a class of steroid hormones that are synthesized by the adrenal cortex of vertebrates and have anti-inflammatory activity

glycogen [ˈglaɪkəʊdʒən]　a polysaccharide, composed of glucose isomers, that is the principal carbohydrate stored by the animal body and is readily converted to glucose when needed for energy use

graafian follicle [ˈgraːfiən] [ˈfɒlɪkəl]　one of the small vesicles containing a developing ovum in the ovary of placental mammals

hydrocortisone [ˌhaɪdrəʊˈkɔːtɪˌzəʊn]　a steroid hormone, of the adrenal cortex, active in carbohydrate and protein metabolism

hypophysis [haɪˈpɒfɪsɪs]　(pl. hypophyses) pituitary gland

hypothalamus [ˌhaɪpəˈθæləməs]　a basal part of the diencephalon that lies beneath the thalamus on each side, forms the floor of the third ventricle, and includes vital autonomic regulatory centers

infundibulum [ˌɪnfʌnˈdɪbjʊləm]　(pl. infundibula) any funnel-shaped part, especially the stalk connecting the pituitary gland to the base of the brain

insulin [ˈɪnsjʊlɪn]　a substance that most people produce naturally in their body and that controls the level of sugar in their blood

interstitial [ˌɪntəˈstɪʃl]　relating to or situated in the interstices

islets of Langerhans [ˈlɒngəhɒnz]　small groups of endocrine cells in the pancreas that secrete the hormones insulin and glucagon

isthmus [ˈɪsməs] (pl. isthmi) a contracted anatomical part or passage connecting two larger structures or cavities

lacrimal [ˈlækrɪməl] of, relating to, or being glands that produce tears

luteinizing hormone [ˈluːtɪɪnaɪzɪŋ] (LH) a hormone produced by the anterior lobe of the pituitary gland that stimulates ovulation and the development of the corpus luteum in the female and the production of testosterone by the interstitial cells of the testis in the male

melanocyte [ˈmelənəʊˌsaɪt] an epidermal cell that produces melanin

mineralocorticoid [ˌmɪnərələʊˈkɔːrtɪˌkɔɪd] any of a group of corticosteroid hormones, synthesized by the adrenal cortex, that regulate the excretion or reabsorption of sodium and potassium by the kidneys, salivary glands, and sweat glands

neuroglia [njʊəˈrɒɡlɪə] a class of cells in the brain and spinal cord that form a supporting and insulating structure for the neurons

norepinephrine [ˌnɔːrepɪˈnefrɪn] a neurotransmitter that is similar to epinephrine, acts to constrict blood vessels and dilate bronchi, used esp. in medical emergencies to raise blood pressure

osteoclast [ˈɒstɪəʊklæst] a large multinuclear cell formed in bone marrow that is associated with the normal absorption of bone

ovulation [ˌɒvjʊˈleɪʃn] the discharge of a mature ovum from the ovary

parathormone [ˌpærəˈθɔːməʊn] parathyroid hormone

pigmentation [ˌpɪɡmenˈteɪʃn] an excessive deposition of bodily pigment

potassium [pəˈtæsɪəm] a silvery-white metallic element that oxidizes rapidly in the air and whose compounds are used as fertilizer and in special hard glasses

progesterone [prəʊˈdʒestəˌrəʊn] a female steroid sex hormone that is secreted by the corpus luteum to prepare the endometrium for implantation and later by the placenta during pregnancy to prevent rejection of the developing embryo or fetus

prolactin [prəʊˈlæktɪn] a protein hormone of the anterior lobe of the pituitary that induces lactation

prostaglandin [ˌprɒstəˈɡlændɪn] any of a class of unsaturated fatty acids that are involved in the contraction of smooth muscle, the control of inflammation and body temperature, and many other physiological functions

sella turcica [ˈselə] [ˈtəsɪkə] saddlelike bony prominence on the upper surface of the body of the sphenoid bone, constituting the middle part of the butterfly-shaped middle cranial fossa

somatotropin [ˌsəʊmətəˈtrəʊpɪn] (also called growth hormone) a hormone produced by the anterior pituitary gland and promotes growth in humans

sphenoid bone [ˈsfiːnɔɪd] the large butterfly-shaped compound bone at the base of the skull, containing a protective depression for the pituitary gland

sympathetic [ˌsɪmpəˈθetɪk] of or relating to the sympathetic nervous system

testis [ˈtestɪs] (pl. testes) the male gonad or reproductive gland, either of two oval glands located in the scrotum

testosterone [teˈstɒstərəʊn] a hormone that is a hydroxy steroid ketone produced especially by the testes or made synthetically and that is responsible for inducing and maintaining male secondary sex characters

thyrotropin [ˌθaɪrəʊˈtrəʊpɪn] (also called thyroid-stimulating hormone) a peptide hormone synthesized and secreted by the anterior pituitary gland, which regulates the endocrine function of the thyroid gland

thyroxine [θaɪˈrɒksiːn]   a hormone of the thyroid gland that regulates the metabolic rate of the body; preparations of it used for treating hypothyroidism

triiodothyronine [traɪˌaɪədəʊˈθaɪrəniːn]   an amino acid hormone that contains iodine and is secreted by the thyroid gland with thyroxine, to which it has a similar action

tyrosine [ˈtaɪrəsiːn]   a phenolic amino acid that is a precursor of several important substances

uterine [ˈjuːtəraɪn]   of, relating to, occurring in, or affecting the uterus

Task 1

Directions: *Select the letter of the choice that best completes the statement or answers the question.*

(1) Growth hormone is secreted by _____.
   A. the thyroid gland   B. the adrenal gland
   C. the anterior pituitary lobe   D. the posterior pituitary lobe

(2) Which of the following glands functions both as an endocrine gland and an exocrine gland?
   A. The parathyroid gland.   B. The pituitary gland.
   C. The adrenal gland.   D. The pancreas.

(3) The hormone that is responsible for stimulating growth and secretion of ovarian follicles and the production of sperm is _____.
   A. TSH   B. FSH   C. ICSH   D. PRL

(4) The hormones which can stimulate the production of milk from the breasts include _____.
   A. prolactin and oxytocin   B. prolactin and vasopressin
   C. vasopressin and oxytocin   D. estrogen and testosterone

(5) The hormones which can regulate the calcium level in the bloodstream include _____.
   A. thyroxin and triiodothyronine   B. TSH and calcitonin
   C. calcitonin and parathormone   D. corticotropin and progesterone

(6) The hormones that prepare us to fight or flee are _____.
   A. aldosterone and renin   B. epinephrine and norepinephrine
   C. cortisol and corticoid   D. thyroxine and triiodothyronine

(7) The thyroid _____.
   A. has a rich blood supply   B. secrets more T3 than T4
   C. produces four hormones   D. is a bean-shaped organ

(8) All of the following are hormones of the anterior pituitary EXCEPT the_____.
   A. growth hormone (GH)   B. follicle-stimulating hormone (FSH)
   C. parathyroid hormone (PTH)   D. thyroid-stimulating hormone (TSH)

(9) The secretions of the endocrine glands are called_____.
   A. enzymes   B. sera   C. lymph   D. hormones

(10) Mineralocorticoids_____.

A. are produced in the adrenal cortex

B. are steroid hormones

C. help regulate the homeostasis of sodium and potassium

D. all of the above

Task 2

Directions: *Label the organs of the endocrine system.*

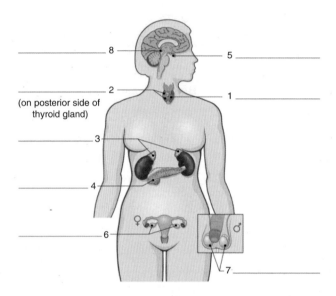

Task 3

Directions: *Fill in the following table based on the text above or relevant information from the Internet and then talk about the the endocrine system.*

Structure	Function
(1) pineal gland	
(2) hypothalamus	
(3) pituitary gland	
(4) parathyroid gland	
(5) thyroid gland	
(6) thymus	
(7) adrenal gland	
(8) pancreas	
(9) ovary	
(10) testicle	

Task 4

Directions: *Match each of the following terms in Column A with its definition in Column B.*

A	B
(1) adrenal cortex	A. outer section (cortex) of each adrenal gland; secretes cortisol, aldosterone, and sex hormones
(2) anterior pituitary	B. pancreatic endocrine cells
(3) islets	C. gland that releases oxytocin
(4) epinephrine	D. male hormone secreted by the testes and to a lesser extent by the adrenal cortex
(5) adrenal medulla	E. somatotropin
(6) androgen	F. gland that secretes ACTH
(7) posterior pituitary	G. steroid hormone secreted by the adrenal cortex, regulating glucose, fat, and protein metabolism
(8) glucocorticoid	H. cavity in the skull that contains the pituitary gland
(9) sella turcica	I. inner section (medulla) of each adrenal gland, secreting epinephrine and norepinephrine
(10) growth hormone	J. hormone produced by the adrenal medulla

Medical Terminology

Roots	Terminology	Term Analysis	Definition
gland			
aden(o) [ˈædɪnəʊ]	adenoma [ˌædɪˈnəʊmə] adenopathy [ˌædɪˈnɒpəθi]	path(o)=disease	
secrete			
crin(o) [ˈkrɪnəʊ]	endocrinologist [ˌendəʊkrɪˈnɒlədʒɪst] exocrine [ˈeksəʊkraɪn]	endo-=inside, within -ist=practitioner of a profession exo-=out	
secret(o) [ˌsɪˈkriːtəʊ]	secretodermatosis [sɪˌkriːtəʊ͵dɜːməˈtəʊsɪs] hypersecretion [ˌhaɪpəsɪˈkriːʃən]	dermat(o)=skin hyper-=above, excessive, beyond	
hormone			
hormon(o) [ˈhɔːmənəʊ]	hormonagogue [hɔːˈmənəgɒg] hormonopoiesis [hɔːmənəpɔɪˈiːsɪs]	agog= denoting a substance that stimulates the secretion of something -poiesis = indicating the act of making or producing something specified	

(to be continued)

pineal gland			
pineal(o) [ˈpɪnɪələʊ]	pineal [ˈpɪnɪəl] pinealoma [ˌpɪnɪəˈləʊmə]		
pituitary gland			
pituit(o) [pɪˈtjuːɪtəʊ]	pituitectomy [pɪˌtjuːɪˈtektəmɪ] pituitarism [pɪˈtjuːɪtərɪzəm]		
thyroid gland			
thyr(o) [ˈθaɪrəʊ]	thyroglobulin [ˌθaɪrɒˈglɒbjʊlɪn] thyrotoxicosis [ˌθaɪrɒˌtɒksɪˈkəʊsɪs] thyroiditis [ˌθaɪrɔɪˈdaɪtɪs] hyperparathyroidism [haɪpəˌpærəˈθaɪrɔɪdɪzm]		
thymus gland			
thym(o) [ˈθaɪməʊ]	euthymism [juːˈθaɪmɪzəm] prothymocyte [prəʊˈθaɪməʊsaɪt]	eu-=good, normal	
pancreas			
pancre(o) [ˈpæŋkrɪəʊ] pancreat(o) [ˈpæŋkrɪətəʊ]	pancrealgia [pæŋkrɪˈældʒɪə] pancreatolysis [pæŋkrɪəˈtɒləsɪs] peripancreatitis [ˌperɪˌpæŋkrɪəˈtaɪtɪs]	alg(o)=pain lys(o)=dissolving, destruction peri-=around	
island, pancreatic islet			
insul(o) [ˈɪnsjʊləʊ]	insulinase [ˈɪnsjʊlɪneɪs] insulinoma [ˌɪnsjʊlɪˈnəʊmə]	-ase=enzyme	
sex gland			
gonad(o) [ˈgɒnədəʊ]	gonadoblastoma [gɒnədəʊblæsˈtəʊmə] gonadotropin [ˌgɒnədəʊˈtrəʊpɪn]	blast(o)=bud,sprout, embryo, formative cells or cell layer trop(o)=acting upon; stimulating	
ovary			

(to be continued)

ovari(o) [əʊˈveərɪəʊ]	ovariohysterectomy [əʊˌveərɪəʊˌhɪstəˈrektəmɪ] ovariorrhaphy [əʊvərɪˈɒrəfɪ]	hyster(o)=womb, uterus -rrhaphy= suture	
testis			
test(o) [ˈtestəʊ]	testitis [tesˈtaɪtɪs] testosterone [tesˈtɒstərəʊn]	-one= ketone	
iodine			
iodi [ˈaɪədɪ]	iodimetry [aɪəˈdɪmɪtrɪ]	metr(o)=measure	
iod(o) [ˈaɪəʊdəʊ]	triiodothyronine [ˌtraɪˌaɪədəʊˈθaɪrɒniːn] tetraiodothyronine [tetrəˌaɪədəʊˈθaɪrɒniːn]	tri-=three tetra-=four	
male			
andr(o) [ˈændrəʊ]	androgen [ˈændrɒdʒən] androsterone [ænˈdrɒstərəʊn]		
female			
estr(o) [ˈestrəʊ]	estradiol [ˌestrəˈdaɪəl] estrogen [ˈestrɒdʒən]	di-=two -ol=an alcohol or a phenol	
sugar			
gluc(o) [ˈgluːkəʊ]	glucocorticoid [ˌgluːkɒˈkɔːtɪkɔɪd] glucagon [ˈgluːkəgɒn]	-oid=indicating likeness, resemblance, or similarity ag-=push forward, put in motion; stir up; excite, urge	
glyc(o) [ˈglaɪkəʊ]	hyperglycemia [ˌhaɪpəglaɪˈsɪmɪə] glycogenolysis [ˌglaɪkɒdʒəˈnɔːlɪsɪs]		
acting upon, stimulating			
trop(o) [ˈtrɒpəʊ]	adrenocorticotropin [əˌdriːnəʊˌkɔːtɪkəʊˈtrɒpɪn] somatotropin [ˌsəʊmətɒˈtrəʊpɪn]	cortic(o)=cortex somat(o)=body	
nourishment, development			

(to be continued)

troph(o) [ˈtrɒfəʊ]	dystrophy [ˈdɪstrəfi] myatrophy [maɪˈætrəfi]	dys-=abnormal, difficult, bad, impaired my(o)=muscle	
steroid			
ster(o) [ˈstɒrəʊ]	corticosteroid [ˌkɔːtɪkəʊˈstɪərɔɪd] hypercholesteremia [ˌhaɪpəkəˌlestəˈriːmɪə]	-oid=resemblance to, equivalent to chol(o)=gall, bile	
mucus			
myx(o) [ˈmɪksəʊ]	myxadenitis [ˌmɪksædɪˈnaɪtɪs] myxedema [ˌmɪksɪˈdiːmə]		
extremity of the body			
acro [ˈækrəʊ]	acromegaly [ˌækrəʊˈmegəli] acrodynia [ˌækrəʊˈdɪnɪə]	megal(o)=enlargement -odynia=pain	

Vocabulary Study

Task 1

Directions: *Match the following terms with the appropriate meanings and underline the strong part of each word where there are two or more syllables.*

(1) thymoma
(2) hyperparathyroidism
(3) adrenopathy
(4) thyroidectomy
(5) myxedema

A. removal of the thyroid gland
B. tumor of the thymus gland
C. increased secretion of parathyroid hormone
D. decreased activity of the thyroid gland in adults
E. disease of the adrenal glands

(6) gonadotropin
(7) adenoma
(8) hyperthyroidism
(9) acromegaly
(10) thyroiditis

A. disorder that results from excess growth hormone
B. overactivity of the thyroid gland
C. a hormone that stimulates the growth and activity of the gonads
D. inflammation of the thyroid gland
E. neoplasm of a gland

Task 2

Directions: *Fill in the blanks with appropriate words for body parts.*

(1) Hypogonadism is a condition caused by undersecretion of the _____.

(2) Adrenomegaly refers to enlargement of the _____.

(3) Euthymism is the state of having normal _____ function.

(4) Surgical removal of the_____ is termed parathyroidectomy.

(5) Pinealoma means the tumor of the _____.

(6) Adenopathy means a diseased condition of a _____.

(7) Hypopituitarism is a condition caused by underactivity of the _____.

(8) Pancreatolysis refers to the destruction of the _____.

(9) A person who has ovariorrhaphy underwent surgical suture of the _____.

(10) When a testectomy is performed, the _____ is removed (or excised).

Task 3

Directions: *Write a word for each of the following definitions using the word parts provided.*

thyr(o)	calc(o)	-osis	gonad(o)	hypo-	
-emia	-ism	toxic(o)	pancreat(o)	-ectomy	-oid

(1) abnormal condition (poison) of the thyroid gland _____

(2) removal of the pancreas _____

(3) condition of deficiency or underdevelopment of the sex organs _____

(4) deficiency of calcium in the blood _____

(5) removal of the thyroid gland _____

-ic	gen	log(o)	glyc(o)	-emia	-ist
hyper	andro	endo	crin(o)	estr(o)	-e

(6) pertaining to producing female characteristics _____

(7) excessive sugar in the blood _____

(8) any steroid hormone producing male characteristics _____

(9) specialist in the study of hormone disorders _____

(10) connected with the internal or hormonal secretion of a ductless gland _____

-al	trop(o)	adren(o)	dys	-in	-y
troph(o)	cortic(o)	ster(o)	-oid	insul(o)	

(11) a hormone that acts on cells of the adrenal cortex, causing them to produce male sex hormones and hormones that control water and mineral balance in the body _____

(12) abnormal development or growth of a tissue or organ, usually resulting from nutritional deficiency _____

(13) a substance that most people produce naturally in their body and that controls the level of sugar in their blood _____

(14) a steroid produced by the cortex of the suprarenal gland _____

(15) pertaining to or arising from the adrenal cortex _____

Case Study 8-1

Cushing's Syndrome in a Child

A 4 years old boy presented with complaints of excessive weight gain of 5 months duration and increased frequency of micturition and appearance of body hair for 4 months. There was no history of any other illness, medication or steroid intake. The child was first born at term by normal vaginal delivery and birth weight of 3 kg. Physical examination revealed a chubby boy with moon face, buffalo hump, protruding abdomen, increased body hair and appearance of coarse pubic hair. His intelligent quotient was appropriate for his age and sex. His younger sibling was in good health and other family members did not have any metabolic or similar problems. The patient's body length was 92 cm, weight 20 kg, and BMI was 23.6. His blood pressure on right arm in lying position was 138/76mm Hg.

Cushing's syndrome is a rare entity in children. Adrenal tumor is the common cause of this syndrome in young children, whereas, iatrogenic causes are more common among older children. This 4-year-old male child was diagnosed with Cushing's syndrome due to a right adrenal adenoma; the child presented with obesity and increase distribution of body hair. After thorough investigation and control of hypertension and dyselectrolytemia, right adrenalectomy was performed. The patient had good clinical recovery with weight loss and biochemical resolution of Cushing's syndrome.

Task 4

Directions: *Select the best answer to the question or the statement based on the information provided in the case of Cushing's syndrome.*

(1) Which of the following could NOT be what the patient complained of?
   A. I have put on many kilos.   B. I take a leak at short intervals.
   C. My appetite is very poor.   D. Body hair can be observed.

(2) Which one is mentioned in the patient's history EXCEPT _____.

    A. other illnesses   B. surgery   C. medications   D. steroid intake

(3) The patient was born by _____.

    A. postdatc gcstation   B. premature delivery

    C. post-term birth   D. full-term pregnancy

(4) The reference of patient's younger sibling and other family members tells _____.

    A. personal history   B. history of present illness

    C. the family history   D. the social history

(5) Which is NOT manifested in the patient with Cushing's syndrome?

    A. Concentric obesity. B. Hirsutism.   C. Normal IQ.   D. Anorexia.

(6) The underlined word "protruding" means _____.

    A. flat   B. bulging   C. recessed   D. circled

(7) Cushing's syndrome is rare in _____.

    A. children   B. adults   C. elderly people   D. middle-aged people

(8) The patient was inflicted by Cushing's syndrome because of _____.

    A. obesity   B. hairy body

    C. the tumor in his adrenal gland   D. congenital factors

(9) The term iatrogenic means _____.

    A. induced in a patient by the treatment   B. induced in a patient by the environment

    C. induced in a patient by virus   D. induced in a patient by bacteria

(10) Before recovery, the patient underwent several procedures EXCEPT _____.

    A. thorough investigation   B. control of hypertension and dyselectrolytemia

    C. surgical excision of the adrenal gland   D. surgical repair of the adrenal gland

Case Study 8-2

Parathyroidectomy

The case pertains to a 42-year-old Caucasian female patient, who was admitted in our department due to general weakness, along with incidents of vague abdominal pain for the past 8 months. Her medical history included 2 Cesarean sections, and she was a periodical smoker. Physical examination was proven unremarkable.

A complete laboratory scan was performed, which demonstrated normal hematocrit and hemoglobin values. Her thyroid hormones revealed an euthyroid state, with TSH, T3 and T4 being within normal limits. Parathormone was 151 pg/mL while serum calcium was detected at the highest normal levels for our laboratory (10.4 mg/dL with a normal range of 8.1–10.5 mg/dL), thus setting the basis for the diagnosis of normocalcemic hyperparathyroidism. Rest of her biochemistry results was insignificant.

An ultrasound scan of her neck revealed a normal sized thyroid gland, while an enlarged parathyroid was located on the left lower side of her cervical region, with its dimensions approximately 3×2 cm. Further examination with 99 m Tc-MIBI parathyroid scintigraphy depicted large concentrations of radiotracer on the same location, signifying a possible parathyroid adenoma as the cause of her hyperparathyroidism (Fig. 1). After signing written consent, the patient was taken to the operating room.

Resection of the giant gland was performed by a general surgeon experienced in thyroid surgery through implementation of minimal invasive parathyroidectomy (MIP). A small left-sided thyroid incision was performed, approximately 2 cm in length. After lateral retraction of the sternothyroid muscle and manipulation of the left thyroid lobe, the gross parathyroid adenoma was located, attached on the posterior side of the left lower lobe of her thyroid (Fig. 2). Careful resection of the gland was performed with identification of the left recurrent laryngeal nerve. The excised specimen was sent for pathologic examination, which was indeed significant for a giant 3 × 2 cm parathyroid adenoma (Fig. 3).

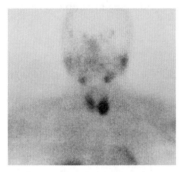

Figure 1. 99 m Tc-MIBI parathyroid scintigraphy demonstrated increased radiotracer absorption from the lower left parathyroid gland.

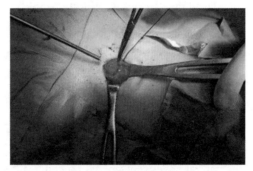

Figure 2. A giant parathyroid adenoma resected through implementation of minimally invasive parathyroidectomy. The gland was removed through a small left-sided thyroid incision.

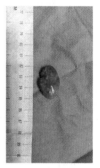

Figure 3. Excised specimen of a giant 3 × 2 cm parathyroid adenoma

The postoperative period was uneventful for the patient, with a slight decline in calcium (9.5 mg/dL), and her parathormone (PTH) levels returned within normal limits approximately 8 hours after surgery. She was discharged on the next day, while at 3 month follow up she reported no further symptoms.

Task 5

Directions: *Write a word or phrase from the case study that means the same as each of the following.*

(1) a surgical incision through the abdominal wall and uterus, performed to deliver a fetus

(2) the red substance in blood, which combines with oxygen and carries it around the body

(3) the thyroid gland that functions normally

(4) the process of examining the body by means of sight, touch, percussion, or auscultation to diagnose disease or verify fitness

(5) the fluid portion of the blood obtained after removal of the fibrin clot and blood cells, distinguished from the plasma in circulating blood

(6) a diagnostic method of examining internal organs using high-frequency sound waves

(7) of or pertaining to the sternum and the thyroid cartilage

(8) to formally terminate a person's care in and release them from a hospital or healthcare facility

(9) surgical removal of all or part of an organ, tissue, or structure

(10) a diagnostic technique using a radioactive tracer and scintillation counter for producing pictures of internal parts of the body

Medical Term Extension

Common Abbreviations in Medicine

The healthcare field is full of technical terminology, including a number of medical abbreviations that are used to complete patient charts, write prescriptions, communicate general needs and bill for services. Being able to access a medical abbreviation list can help you take control of your healthcare needs.

Abbreviations to know
as a medical student

p/w: presents with	VSS: vital signs stable
c/o: complains of	WNL: within normal limits
s/p: status post	I&O: intake and output
d/c: discharge	ASA: aspirin
n/v: nausea and vomiting	NTG: nitroglycerin
s/s: signs and symptoms	Abx: antibiotics
f/u: follow up	CHF: congestive heart failure
bx: biopsy	HTN: hypertension
dx: diagnosis	GCS: Glasgow Coma Scale
fx: fracture	MVA: motor vehicle accident
rx: prescription	PNA: pneumonia
tx: treatment	PTX: pneumothorax
QD: every day	HA: headache
BID: 2x per day	CA: cancer
TID: 3x per day	CXR: chest x-ray
QID: 4x per day	DOE: dyspnea on exertion
PRN: as needed	SOB: shortness of breath
QH: every hour	DTs: delirium tremens
Q3H: every 3 hours	EOM: extraocular muscles
STAT: immediately	US: ultrasound
NPO: nothing by mouth	DNR: do not resuscitate
gtt: drops (IV drip)	DNI: do not intubate
OTC: over the counter	M&M: morbidity and mortality

It's always advisable to consult with your doctor, nurse, pharmacist, or other medical professional about any and all medical terminology that's confusing or unclear. Only those within the medical field can truly decipher the multitude of abbreviations in the industry.

Task 6

Directions: *Write out the full form of each of the following abbreviations. The first one has been done for you as an example.*

ADH: antidiuretic hormone

(1) CT _____ (2) DTaP _____

(3) DM _____ (4) mm Hg _____

(5) ECG (EKG) _____ (6) RBC _____

(7) MS _____ (8) LP _____

(9) HIV _____ (10) ICU _____

Writing

Common Errors in EMP Writing

"...Your paper has been identified as requiring English language copy editing. Note that your paper will not be accepted for publication unless this editing has taken place. Please seek the help of a native English speaker, a specialist English language copy editor or any organization who also provide this service. Please comment on who has helped you with this in your Response to Reviewers letter when submitting your revised paper..."

——from a letter of reviews

According to Peter Thrower, Editor-in-Chief of Carbon, one of the top reasons for rejection is poor language comprehension. Incorrect usage of words, spelling and grammar errors, and flaws in sentence construction can spoil even the greatest research, which makes editing a crucial element in good scientific writing.

Before you proceed to submission you are supposed to ask yourself these questions about language quality.

☆ Is my manuscript free of spelling and grammatical mistakes?
☆ Am I using the right terminology?

☆ Does my paper reflect intelligible word choices, structured sentences, and a logical flow of information?

☆ Is the language used appropriate for scientific literature?

To be considered submission-ready, scientific writing must have the correct use of punctuation, fonts, abbreviations, and grammar among other language guidelines. A second look and in-depth review is required and recommended to help enhance the readability of the manuscript and impress the journal editor, reviewer, and reader. All aspects such as sentence structure, grammar, word choice, style, logic and flow should be improved, if necessary, so as to create a polished well-written manuscript.

The following will be groups of examples of common errors in EMP writing. The revised version and comment are sometimes provided to illustrate how copyediting works and why so.

About Words

Misspelled words in sciences distract and annoy the reader. The credibility of your work hinges on the proper use of the language. Every document that leaves the writer's desk must have undergone careful screening for spelling errors, both by the author/editor and the spell checker. A mixture of American and British spelling within any one document is both confusing and annoying to the reader. If you have the choice, use either American or British spelling, but do so consistently. Keep your target audience in mind (European versus international). If language requirements are defined (e.g., company-internal conventions, journal house style, publishers' requirements), use the given spelling rules consistently. For example:

All histological and histopathologic findings from the foetuses confirmed the presence of multiple oedemas.

In American research report, it should be written as:

All histologic and histopathologic findings from the fetuses confirmed the presence of multiple edemas.

Another example:

This was a single-center, placebo-controlled study to determine the effects of the LH-RH analog on estrogen levels in a pediatric population with central precocious puberty.

In European clinical study, it should be written as:

This was a single-centre, placebo-controlled study to determine the effects of the LH-RH analogue on oestrogen levels in a paediatric population with central precocious puberty.

In American English, "al" omitted in adjectives such as "histological"; "e" for "oe" in "foetuses" and "oedemas".

In European English / British English, "centre" rather than "center"; "analogue" rather than "analog"; "oe" for "e" in "estrogen"; "ae" for "e" in "pediatric".

Numbers play an important role in scientific communication. Spell out numbers at the beginning of a sentence. With very large numbers, rearrange the sentence in such a way that the number is no longer at the beginning. Always use numerals if a unit of measurement follows (e.g., 3 mL, 9 h, 5 min). In a series, use numerals if any number in the series is 10 or larger (e.g., In total, 2 monkeys, 5 rabbits, and 12 rats were used). If two numbers appear back to back, write one out (e.g., ten 20-mg doses).

> Sales were substantially higher in 2013 than last year (i.e., 1.2×10^9 units versus 0.8×10^9 units sold in 2012).
>
> Serious adverse events occurred in 5 (10%) patients. Of the 1278 patients participating, 37 (2.9%) did not respond to treatment.

Capitalized words in science are either proper nouns, key words in titles, or first words of sentences.

> **Pharmacokinetic** Parameters of the Parent Compound and the Three Metabolites in Plasma of Rats, Rabbits, and Monkeys
> As indicated, Table 5 summarizes the demographic data. For individual data consult Appendix 2.

About Tense

Proper use of tense in scientific documents derives from scientific ethics, i.e., we owe it to the scientific community to declare, by the choice of tense, whether we report established facts or new, previously unpublished data. When a scientific paper has been published in a primary journal (i.e., a journal that publishes only original data), the information communicated becomes "established knowledge". This definition often creates heated discussion among my students as they point out, quite rightly, that so many a published "fact" will prove untrue in subsequent studies. In this respect, "established knowledge" occasionally turns out to be a transient phenomenon. Nonetheless, validly published findings are regarded as "knowledge" as long as the findings have not been challenged or even disproved elsewhere.

Established knowledge

> HIV infection is highly prevalent in African countries [12].

Your own new finding

> Inhibition of the enzyme resulted in much higher plasma levels of the parent drug.

When referring to your finding after its publication

> Inhibition of the enzyme results in much higher plasma levels of the parent drug [2].

Thus, the rule to remember is this: Report established knowledge in the present tense but new, previously unpublished findings (including your own results) in the past tense.

Next shows the tense appropriate in a specific context or section of a scientific manuscript.

Context of section	Appropriate tense
Established knowledge, previous results, etc.	Present tense
Methods, materials used, and results	Past tense
Description of tables and figures	Present tense, e.g., Table 5 shows…; Figure 2 illustrates…
Attribution	Past tense, e.g., Jones et al. reported that…; Davies found…

About Parallelism

Confused scientific writing often comes about by erroneously joining sentences, clauses, or even single terms. The resulting incoherence is called "nonparallelism." I would argue that nonparallelism is, indeed, responsible for many errors, some of which are serious enough to lead the reader to draw the wrong conclusions. Nonparallel statements often come about because we think faster than we write or because we expect the reader to deduce the correct message from our statements although the text is unclear. Another reason for the many nonparallel sentences in science is carelessness, an attitude grossly incompatible with the enormous precision we exercise when doing scientific work. Please bear in mind that it is unfair to the readers of our paper to let them guess what we were trying to say.

Nonparallel statements may occur on all levels of a sentence, for example when joining nouns, verbs, modifiers, prepositional phrases, or entire sentences. The joining words are called conjunctions, and these may be of the coordinating or subordinating type. Coordinating conjunctions join terms that are equals, whereas subordinating conjunctions show inequality or a relationship of dependence or limitation. Both types of conjunctions may be involved in nonparallel constructions.

Incorrect

> A small volume of water was added to the mixture and the samples incubated for 24 h.

Correct

> A small volume of water was added to the mixture, and the samples were incubated for 24 h.

Incorrect

> Incubation times were 2 h, 6 h, and 12 h, respectively.

Correct

> Incubation times for experiments 1, 2, and 3 were 2 h, 6 h, and 12 h, respectively.

Incorrect

> We developed this novel laxative for patients with hemorrhoids, anal fissures, and after surgery.

Correct

> We developed this novel laxative for patients with hemorrhoids and anal fissures, and for patients who have undergone surgery.

About Sequence

For a sentence to make sense, the words must be presented in a logical sequence. If the words are not in reasonable order, the result can be ridiculous, as shown below:

Confusing syntax

> We selected an investigator with considerable expertise in the field called Mike Miller.

Confusing syntax

> The study involved a small group of children in a Swiss children's hospital with juvenile diabetes.

Clear syntax

> We selected an investigator called Mike Miller who has considerable expertise in the field.

Clear syntax

> The study involved a small group of children with juvenile diabetes in a Swiss children's hospital.

Grammatically correct

> It is the investigator's duty to inform the patient fully before initiating the therapy.

Preferred because the meaning is clearer

> It is the investigator's duty to fully inform the patient before initiating the therapy.

About Dangling

Unfortunately, verbal phrase danglers are abundant in scientific reporting. They contribute substantially to misleading messages and confused writing. In most cases, the problem arises from a lack of logical thinking or poor word order. Many danglers escape the author's and/or editor's attention because the readers' brains may deduce the intended message, disregarding the fact that the sentence says something totally different. Needless to say, guesswork is incompatible with science, and it is unacceptable to let our readers guess what we have meant to say.

Let us consider an example:

Incorrect because of dangling participle

> Structured into various sections, the readers of this review can choose the topic of primary interest.

Correct

> The review is structured into various sections, which allows the readers to choose the topic of primary interest.

Incorrect because of dangling participle

> Based on experience, microsomal preparations are more useful than hepatocytes.

Correct

> Experience shows that microsomal preparations are more useful than hepatocytes.

Better because active

> We consider microsomal preparations more useful than hepatocytes.

Task 1

Directions: *The passage below needs to be corrected with one error in each line. You should point out the mistake as well as the way to correct it.*

Example:

I have a English book.   <u>an</u>

> It was the second admision of the 61-year-old man
> who complained of the chronical morning cough
> in 10 years' duration. He stated the cough is productive
> with the whitish-yellow sputa. And several month ago,
> a cough somewhat differently from before developed
> and became progressive worse. One month ago, he stopped
> smoking. Then the cough seemed to have been improved.
> But three weeks ago, he noticed blood-tinge sputum. Two
> weeks before admission, he developed sharp stabbing pain
> in the left-sided chest
> which is associating with somewhat but later actual
> pleuritic nature for 48 hours.

_____
_____
_____
_____
_____
_____
_____
_____

Task 2

Directions: *The following sentences contain one error each. Proofread and correct them carefully by crossing out the wrong places and writing down the correct versions on the answer sheet.*

(1) Notable, the bioelectrical impedance cell culture platforms are fully characterized and the findings are confirmed with those of optical microscopy and electrochemical (including pH) assays.

(2) The nNOS is a Ca^{2+}-dependent constitutive synthase, and its activity is strictly regulated by N-methyl-D-aspartate receptor (NMDAR)-mediated increase in the concentration of intracellular Ca^{2+}.

(3) Moreover, a study by Hashimoto and colleagues demonstrated that the accumulation of CAPON in neurons induce an obviously high level of phosphorylated, insoluble tau protein and neuronal cell death, suggesting that CAPON is a novel tau-binding protein.

(4) Blood testing including calcium, phosphorus, alkaline phosphatase, and 25-hydroxy vitamin D (25-(OH)D) and plasma VPA level were measured at 1-to-3-month intervals.

(5) A 53-year-old man diagnosed by annuloaortic ectasia (66 mm in root diameter) and severe AR with Marfan syndrome underwent modified Bentall procedure using valved graft.

(6) With the understanding of pathophysiology of the disease, we have developed different treatment options to improve the survive rates of CRC patients.

(7) The physical examination was normal.

(8) The presence of cystic or necrotic components were significantly more frequent in PNENs G2 (15/42, 35.7%) than in PNENs G1 (5/39, 12.8%, P=0.017).

(9) A more convergent distribution of mutations was observed in the Chinese cohort (P-value=0.012) compared with scattered mutations in Caucasians LUAD.

(10) The patient was performed an operation yesterday.

(11) The composition of VOCs were analyzed by GC-MS (Trace 1310/ISQ-LT, Thermo Scientific, USA).

(12) Previous studies demonstrated that family history of cervical cancer was associated with cervical cancer risk, supporting the critical role of genetic susceptibility in cervical carcinogenesis.

(13) A prior study showed that MALAT-1 expression was upregulated in cervical cancer cells compared with normal cells.

(14) Individuals with 3—4 unfavorable alleles had 18% increased odds of having cervical cancer than those with 0—1 unfavorable allele.

(15) We further performed stratified analysis by age, menarche age, parity, menopausal status.

(16) The assessment of the ulnar nerve is therefore preferred over the facial nerve, because electricity may excite the facial muscles directly and make them contract even though the neuromuscular junction has been blocked completely.

(17) Title: Preliminary experience in high dose methotrexate therapy in acute lymphocytic leukemia.

(18) Data were summarized as mean ±SD.

(19) A patient had a fever of 39.5℃ .

(20) The tissue was minced and the samples incubated.